haviors."—Laura Fraser, author of *Losing It: America's Obsession with Weight and the Industry that Feeds it*

"[Waterhouse] deals with a rarely discussed topic: how a mother's dysfunctional eating habits are frequently passed on to and imitated by their daughters. These patterns lead to adverse health effects for both generations. This important book will lift the veil that clouds this issue and provide all mothers and daughters with helpful and effective solutions to this problem."—Susan M. Lark, M.D., author of *Self-Help for PMS* and *Self-Help for Menopause*

"A very practical, readable, eye-opening book that can revolutionize the way women relate to their bodies, their food, their daughters, and each other."—Adele Faber, co-author of *How to Talk so Kids Will Listen & Listen so Kids Will Talk*

"Debra Waterhouse has created a valuable resource for my groups of Mothers of Daughters with Eating Disorders! I've added *Like Mother, Like Daughter* to my recommended reading list."—Avis Rumney, M.A., MFCC, eating disorders specialist and author of *Dying to Please: Anorexia Nervosa and Its Cure*

"This is an important and comprehensive book about the linkage between childhood experiences and adult dieting obsessions. The reader is gracefully introduced to the sociology, psychology, and research literature on mothers' and daughters' dieting and food addictions. The author offers insights on why 'real women don't diet.' Don't misplace this book."—Michael J. Maloney, M.D., director of the Eating Disorders Clinic, Children's Hospital, and University of Ohio Krug Associate Professor of Psychiatry and Pediatrics

"Written in a lively, engaging style, *Like Mother, Like Daughter* offers women creative and constructive solutions to free them from the tyranny of dieting, disordered eating, and body dissatisfaction. Waterhouse explains the danger in the late twentieth-century tradition of mothers handing down diets to their daughters, without indicting mothers—how refreshing! This diet-breaking book will liberate women of all generations from our inherited body hatred and will return control of our bodies to us. Thank you, Debra Waterhouse."—Margo Maine, Ph.D., director of the Eating Disorders Institute of Living, author of *Father Hunger: Fathers, Daughters and Food*, president of Eating Disorders Awareness & Prevention.

"Debra Waterhouse again masterfully dispels the myths about dieting *and* offers us crucial insight into the family food lineage. A "must read" for *every* mother and daughter!"—Jeanne and Don Elium, authors of *Raising a Daughter, Raising a Son*, and *Raising a Family*

"I highly recommend this book to all women, their daughters, and to the men who love them. . . . In this book, Debra reveals how these subtle pressures to achieve unrealistic weights are inadvertently passed from mother to daughter and, more importantly, how to break the cycle, recapture the pride, and pass down an empowering torch to the next generation."—Elizabeth Somer, M.D., R.D., author of *Food & Mood* and *Nutrition for Women*

"Personal and motivating, a must-read for mothers and daughters who seek to better understand their relationship with food."—Catherine Christie, Ph.D., R.D., president of Nutrition Associates, Inc.

"Well-researched and written with the flair that Waterhouse created in her previous best-sellers. *Like Mother, Like Daughter* belongs in every resource library and center that reaches out to women of all ages."—Judith Briles, Ph.D., editor of *The Woman's Voice*, author of *Gender Traps* and *The Confidence Factor*

"American women have been waiting to hear this message for twenty years."—Debbie Herlax-Durga, owner, designer, Fitness P.T.

Also by Debra Waterhouse, MPH, RD

Why Women Need Chocolate:
How to Get the Body You Want by Eating the Foods You Crave

Outsmarting the Female Fat Cell:
The First Weight-Control Program Designed
Specifically for Women

LIKE MOTHER, LIKE DAUGHTER

How women are influenced by their

mothers' relationship with food

—and how to break the pattern

DEBRA WATERHOUSE, MPH, RD

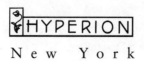

New York

The advice in this book is not intended for persons with chronic illnesses or other conditions that may be worsened by an unsupervised eating program. The recommendations are not intended to replace or conflict with advice given to you by your physician, pediatrician, or other health professional, and we recommend that you do consult with your physician.

Except for those who have given the author permission to use their names, all names in this book have been changed. In some cases, composite accounts have been created based on the author's professional experience.

Copyright © 1997, Debra Waterhouse, MPH, RD

Page 155—Reprinted with permission, *Tufts University Diet & Nutrition Letter*.

Page 114–115—Researched by John Hastings. Adapted from *Health*, © 1992.

Page 116—Reprinted by permission of Elsevier Science, Inc., from "Perceptions of Weight and Attitudes Toward Eating in Early Adolescent Girls," by Elissa Koff, Ph.D., *Journal of Adolescent Health Care*, Volume 12, Number 4, pages 307–310. Copyright © 1991 by the Society for Adolescent Medicine.

p. 122—Reprinted with permission from *The I Hate to Diet Dictionary* by Sandra Bergeson. Copyright © 1984 by Turnbull & Willoughby Pub., Inc.

Library of Congress Cataloging-in-Publication Data
Waterhouse, Debra.
   Like mother, like daughter : how women are influenced by their mothers' relationship with food—and how to break the pattern / Debra Waterhouse.—1st ed.
     p.   cm.
   Includes bibliographical references and index.
   ISBN 0-7868-6167-3
   1. Women—Health and hygiene. 2. Mothers and daughters.
  3. Weight loss. 4. Food habits. I. Title.
RA778.W2188 1997
613'.0424—dc20   96–19166
                                      CIP

Book design by Robert Bull Design
FIRST EDITION
10 9 8 7 6 5 4 3 2 1

To my mother
and
her mother
who have passed on a legacy of
female strength, independence, and pride

ACKNOWLEDGMENTS

As I think about the many important people who guided me in the writing of this book, it comes as no surprise that almost all of them are women. My female support system is vital in all I do, and I am grateful to the amazing women whose wisdom and insight contributed greatly to this book—as well as to my life.

Two women in particular, my sister and my editor, deserve the greatest acknowledgment because they have been anchored by my side from start to finish. My sister, Lori Waterhouse Erwin, has reached an unprecedented level of sisterhood and friendship. And my editor, Judith Riven, has risen to an undocumented level of patience, dedication, and leadership.

I will be forever indebted to my sister-in-law, Laura Euphrat, for her daily words of encouragement, but even more so for delivering my first beautiful niece, Christina, and giving me indescribable joy in the midst of my most intense writing.

During the many months I thought of nothing else besides mothers and daughters, my mother-in-law, Laura Manca, continually checked in to make sure that I was taking care of my basic needs, and my mother, Alina Waterhouse, sent her love and positive energy each and every day from 3,000 miles away. Writing this book has given me a deeper appreciation of her love, selflessness, and strength—and has brought me even closer to her.

Many close friends and colleagues donated their valuable time to be my readers. Joyce Filatreau, Stephanie Goulding, RN, Mary Pat Cedarleaf, Michelle Hawkins, Maryann Piacentini, Karen McElhatton, Dr. Elizabeth Markley Holm, RD, and Stephanie Karras, RD, all offered their expertise as mothers, daughters, and/or health professionals. Special appreciation goes to Dr. Dee Tivenan, whose positive influence on this book goes beyond manuscript reading to the foundation of my eating philosophies. I have shared an office with this gifted therapist for over a decade, and through our work together with eating disorder clients and leading women's support groups, she has contributed significantly to my psychological understanding of eating issues and my skills in counseling women.

An immense amount of research went into this book, the extent of which could not have been achieved without Dr. Laura Nathan and Dr. Christine Lafia, sociologists at Mills College and managing partners of Informed Decisions Research, who gave their precious time and enthusiastic spirit to lead my focus groups, or without Amanda and Sarah Kearney, who spent days (months?) in the library doing literature searches, on the computer doing research summaries, and on the phone making follow-up calls. I also extend my sincere thanks to the hundreds of women who participated in my focus groups, answered my questionnaires, and/or took part in my interviews. This book could not have been written without you.

Of course, I wouldn't even be writing this acknowledgment had it not been for my agent, Sandra Dijkstra, who continues to keep me in awe with her unfailing expertise and commitment; her associate, Rita Holm, who consistently makes herself available for my every need; and my publishers, Brian DeFiore and Bob Miller, whose belief in their authors makes them champions in the publishing world.

And as always, loving thanks goes to my supportive husband, Paul Manca, who never once questioned my need to focus on this project at the expense of spending time with him.

CONTENTS

AN IMPORTANT NOTE

TO MOTHERS

After fifteen years of counseling women and more recently interviewing hundreds of mothers and daughters, leading focus groups, and researching over 400 studies for this book, I have come to three important conclusions:

1. The pursuit of thinness through dieting has reached epidemic proportions in *all* female age groups, creating unhealthy food relationships in the vast majority of mothers and daughters.

2. Weight-loss behaviors are so firmly integrated into our daily lives that mothers diet without thinking about it and pass along their weight preoccupations to their daughters without realizing it. By modeling these behaviors and setting the standard for female identity:

   • a mother's dieting history becomes her daughter's dieting future

   • a mother's eating habits are passed on to her daughter

   • a mother's poor body image is mirrored by her daughter

3. When women become aware of how their mothers' relationship with food influenced theirs and how their own eating behaviors and body image are influencing their daughters', they are determined to help themselves and their families achieve a diet-free, body-accepting lifestyle.

My purpose in writing this book is to share with you how I came to these revelations and, more important, to offer you a new approach to eating that will break the chain of destructive patterns and allow you to create a healthier legacy for your family.

In the first chapter, I will alert you to the "trap" of dieting that has imprisoned mothers and daughters of every age and ethnic and economic group since the 1960s. Through a review of alarming research findings and an analysis of your own family, you will discover how the culture of dieting and thinness affected the way your mother raised you and the way you are raising your daughter. Through this important awareness, you will also recognize how the weight-loss methods of your daughter's generation are more drastic and dangerous than those of yours. To give you a glimpse of some of this research, current statistics show that:

- 88% of all mothers have dieted,[1] and 80% of their adolescent daughters have already embarked on their first diet.[2]

- 75% of all mothers "feel" too fat,[3] and 81% of their teenage daughters suffer from this same feeling of weight preoccupation.[4]

- an estimated 60% of all mothers have practiced severe weight-loss attempts through repeated dieting, skipping meals, fasting, laxatives, diuretics, vomiting, and/or excessive exercise. And 80% of their daughters are following in their unhealthy footsteps.

You may find these statistics shocking and disconcerting, but they reflect what is happening or will happen to us and our daughters *unless we free our families from the dieting trap.*

To begin breaking the pattern of destructive eating habits, the next few chapters will help you to identify the many ways you may be teaching unhealthy weight-loss behaviors and body dissatisfaction to your daughter. You may be controlling your daughter's eating habits, restricting her fat and sugar intake, encouraging her to diet, or modeling poor body image. You are your daughter's first female role model and mentor. She is looking to you for validation of her female body. If you are constantly looking for a diet to battle your body fat, she will learn that women are supposed to be at war with their bodies. If you are depriving yourself of food and eating pleasure, she will surmise that women are supposed to undernourish themselves with unsatisfying foods.

Let me assure you that my aim is not to cause blame, guilt, or any other negative reaction. You have been serving as society's messenger, passing along the increasing number of food restrictions and signals of poor body image to your daughter. Since the first super-thin model appeared in the 1960s, the pursuit of thinness has been supported by virtually all segments of society, including the fashion industry, the medical profession, and the media. Today, with the recent rise in obesity, even more emphasis has been placed on food restrictions and dieting. But little information has been given to educate you about how dieting can add to the obesity problem by causing greater weight gain. Thus, in your well-intentioned efforts to ensure a happy, healthy life for your daughter, you may have inadvertently caused her to gain weight and become preoccupied with food. Your current actions are not from lack of care but rather from a lack of knowledge. Chapters 4 through 8 will provide all the necessary knowledge and skills for you to successfully prevent obesity, improve body image, rise above society's restrictive eating rules, and create a new legacy of healthy food relationships.

"Healthy food relationships" may mean something other than what you think. When I first shared the topic of this book with mothers, most of them thought that a healthy mother-daughter food relationship must be about healthy food choices. Their initial response was always similar. "I am very careful about what I eat and what I feed my daughter. I don't have a lot of junk in the house, and I make sure she has a low-fat and low-sugar diet." We are so conditioned to think in terms of "good" and "bad" foods that we presume a "good" mother must serve only fat-free and sugar-free foods.

But that's *not* what *Like Mother, Like Daughter* is about. I believe an overemphasis on "good" foods and "healthy" eating is partially responsible for the recent dieting epidemic and the unhealthy mother-daughter food bond. In this book, you will find minimal information on how you can eat more healthfully but an abundance on how to establish a healthier relationship with food and, therefore, a healthier mother-daughter food relationship. This new relationship will be free of dieting, restriction, control, body dissatisfaction, and guilt—and full of trust, pleasure, satisfaction, and body acceptance.

As you work toward creating a healthier eating legacy for your daughter, you will no doubt reflect on your mother's eating behavior, how it affected you, and how you may be replicating it with your daughter. Just as it is important to understand your influence on your daughter's eating habits, you must also seek to understand your own mother's actions.

Depending on your age and your mother's personal background, her effect on your relationship with food may take one of two forms. She may have been one of the first participants in the pursuit of thinness and, therefore, put you on a diet at an early age, given you your first girdle as a teenager, or cooked you a never-ending menu of diet meals. Or, because of past experiences with food shortages and starvation, she may have disregarded the pursuit of thinness and instead offered you a constant supply of food, encouraged you to gain weight to be "healthy," or forced you to clean your plate.

As I reflect on my former unhealthy relationship with food, I realize that my mother's influence arose from the latter situation. Unlike most young mothers in the 1960s and '70s, she did not diet or encourage me to diet. For her, self-starvation was unthinkable because she had once experienced mass starvation. She was a young girl in Poland when the Nazis confiscated her family's farmhouse and transported her and her family to the terrors of a labor camp. While she has not yet shared with me all of her experiences, what she has shared and what I know of the Holocaust have given me great insight into the woman she is now and the young mother she once was.

My mother is the strongest person I know. She was determined to give my sister and me what she was deprived of as a child: emotional and financial security, independence, educational opportunities—and an abundance of food. Haunted by memories of childhood hunger, she always kept our refrigerator well stocked, cupboards full, and dinner plates overflowing. Her mission was to keep us from becoming malnourished.

Why then, as a teenager, did I undernourish myself and diet down to a figure resembling that of a labor camp victim? Why did

I cause the same pain in myself that my mother tried so desperately to prevent? I have pondered these questions many times and always come up with complex answers. At five foot six inches and ninety-nine pounds, I often wonder if I was trying to *connect* with her relatively unknown and unimaginable past through self-starvation or trying to *disconnect* from her invincible, matriarchal power by refusing to eat. Or was I trying to do both—and thereby achieving the dual goals of identifying with my mother and rebelling against her?

So goes the complicated nature of mother-daughter relationships, finding the balance between identification and individuation. Research has found that this search is often acted out through food (one of the more concrete symbols of the mother) and is compounded by other personality traits. At the backdrop of my personal search was a personality trait that my mother and I both share—perfectionism.

My mother reminds me that I was a perfectionist at birth. As a toddler, every strand of hair had to be exactly in place and every piece of clothing immaculate. In elementary school, I strove to be number one in my class. In high school, my peers called me "Little Miss Perfect" (even today, typing this nickname makes me cringe), and in college, my friends called me "Sally Simmons" to describe my perfect, straight-A, do-good nature at Simmons College. My mother is also a seasoned perfectionist who as a young woman wanted to be the perfect mother with perfect daughters in a perfect house. And I wanted to be the perfect daughter and the perfect student with a perfect body. Like mother, like daughter.

Initially, dieting was my way to achieve a perfect body, but then, as it often does, dieting took on a life of its own. Now as an adult, I realize that my mother could have been a positive role model of healthy, instinctive eating behaviors. She did not and does not restrict foods, nor does she overeat. She eats what she wants, enjoys food, and listens to her body's food messages. Because of her healthy relationship with food, she has always been at a comfortable, healthy weight with a good body image. However, during my developmental years, my own perfectionist tendencies and rebellious, independent nature overrode any positive effect from her modeling a healthy food and body relationship.

Today I fully understand that my mother's determination to nourish me stemmed from infinite love and concern. Society's relentless pressure for thinness may have caused your mother to restrict your food intake and encourage you to diet—again from love and concern. Either way, recognizing the reasons behind our mothers' actions as well as our own contribution to creating an unhealthy legacy will help us to move beyond blame, break the generational chain of disruptive eating patterns, and give our daughters the freedom to respect and feed the bodies they were born with. But we have to respect and feed ours first. Do you?

Right now, if given the choice, would you choose an all-expenses-paid trip around the world or a permanent weight loss of twenty pounds? Would you opt for a job promotion or a body like Cindy Crawford's?

If you have to ponder these questions a bit, don't be too dismayed. Because our society values thinness, we are led to believe that success, power, and happiness come from constricting our bodies and not from setting them free. In fact, a national survey asking similar questions found that 33,000 women were more likely to choose weight loss over career advancement, male relationships, and female friendships.[5] Our culturally driven, misguided goals and priorities have become so universal that there are now many truth-revealing jokes and fables. Here's one that a client told me: A woman finds a magic lantern and a genie appears granting her the one wish of her dreams. Without hesitation, she says "I wish for thin thighs!" In light of world hunger, the homeless, crime, pollution, and environmental decay, the genie is appalled by her wish. Feeling a little guilty, she says "All right then, thin thighs for all women in the world!"

What would be the wish of your dreams?

My professional wish is for *all* women—mothers, daughters, mothers-to-be, grandmothers, aunts, sisters, teachers, health professionals, and community leaders—to wake up to the dangers of this unhealthy legacy of dieting, embrace the diet-free, healthy years ahead, and give the coming generation a full future. My hope is that you will help me in my mission by making the vital transformation to healthier food relationships with both your mother and your daughter.

As you begin reading this book, I encourage you to take the time to laugh a bit and enjoy the process of giving up dieting and the diet mentality. One client said it best when she exclaimed, "My daughter and I have had so much fun living your motto 'Real Women Don't Diet' and going from dieting hell to eating heaven!" I hope that this will become your liberating motto too. Although chronic dieting and body dissatisfaction are serious problems, a sense of humor and an eagerness for knowledge make every step toward a healthier food relationship enjoyable and rewarding.

I wish you, your daughter, and your mother much enjoyment and success in fostering healthier food relationships. You have an opportunity to create a healthy legacy and to ensure its passage to your daughter, granddaughters, great-granddaughters, and all future generations of women.

*Every mother contains her daughter in herself
and every daughter her mother, and every
woman extends backward into her mother
and forward into her daughter.*

—Carl Jung, *The Collected Works*

CHAPTER ONE

THE
GENERATION
TRAP

As *we look* in the mirror at our own reflections, an image of another woman looks back at us: our mother. Whether she is in the same house, in another country, or in the heavens, the connections we share with our mothers can at times astound us as well as comfort us. We know that she has passed along unique biological genes, a long family history, a definition of female identity, and certain personality traits and values that will be with us always.

But as we continue to focus on this mirror reflection, more contemporary mother-daughter similarities start to become apparent. Your eyes may travel down to your thighs with a look of discouragement, feelings of guilt may emerge from last night's chocolate treat, or a renewed vow to start dieting may escape your lips—just like you remember your mother doing a hundred times before. With today's many societal pressures for thinness, the mother-daughter connection now goes far beyond genetics and family history to include deep-rooted food and body issues. As a result, mothers are unwittingly passing along a legacy of unhealthy dieting behaviors and body dissatisfaction to their daughters.

Since the first super-thin model appeared in the 1960s and the first weight-loss clinic opened its doors shortly thereafter, dieting has become a national epidemic and a cornerstone of the mother-daughter bond. After just three generations, the number of dieting adult women has jumped by 300 percent.[1] And the number of dieting girls has risen by a staggering 1,300 percent![2]

For your mother, you, your daughter, and millions of other families, dieting has become an unhappy way of life—and an unhealthy female legacy that knows no boundaries. Healthy-weight women, underweight women, marathon runners, aerobics instructors, and fashion models all report weight worries, as do female celebrities, politicians, nutritionists, physicians, full-time moms, and full-time CEOs. In the pursuit of thinness, one's body weight, occupation, and career success have become irrelevant.

And unfortunately, so has age. Four-year-olds are drinking diet soft drinks; six-year-olds are concerned about how they look in bathing suits; eight-year-olds are weighing themselves every morning; and ten-year-olds are fasting.

Historically, body shape and physical appearance have always been important to women—but *not* to young girls. In the nineteenth century, women wore corsets to shrink their waists, accentuate their hips, and achieve the desired hourglass figure. Some were hospitalized for fainting, cracked ribs, dislodged livers, and collapsed uteruses. A few even went to the extreme of surgically removing their lower ribs to make their waists ever so small. But by the mid-twentieth century, the ideal female figure had been transformed from a curvy hourglass to a curveless test tube. Girdles had long ago replaced corsets, and self-mutilation took on the forms of jaw wiring, stomach stapling, and self-starvation with dieting. Today chronic dieting, fear of fat, and body dissatisfaction are all characteristics of our adolescent daughters. The University of California at San Francisco found that, by age ten, 80 percent are dieting and 60 percent fear weight gain.[3]

Our daughters are not biologically programmed to diet or emotionally predisposed to fear weight gain. These are *learned* behaviors. Daughters learn them from other women, peers, mentors, and the media—*but especially from their mothers.*

- A mother who diets is likely to have a young daughter who diets.
- A mother who diets ten times a year is likely to raise a daughter who diets *more* than ten times a year.

- A mother who is weight preoccupied is likely to bring up her daughter to be weight preoccupied.

Some mothers play an active role by underfeeding their daughters or putting them on diets. Others play a passive role by modeling dietlike behaviors. But if you are one of the 96 percent of all women with weight worries,[4] then you are also worried about your daughter's weight and will unintentionally raise her to have weight worries of her own.

Is your daughter preoccupied with her weight? If she were to look in the mirror, what body and food reflection would she see? What parts of your mother's relationship with food are being passed to her through you, and what parts unique to you are being willed to her?

In your own family as well as in the vast majority of grandmothers, mothers, and daughters today, the ever-increasing pressure for thinness has caused an almost universal transfer of body unhappiness, food fears, restrictive eating habits, and weight struggles—forming a trap of unhealthy food and body relationships that has caught millions of women and girls.

IS YOUR FAMILY CAUGHT IN THE TRAP?

> *My mother started dieting at my age after her third child; I started at age fifteen, half her age—and my daughter is already counting calories at age nine!*
>
> —*Susan, age 29*

When I asked Susan to describe her, her mother's, and her daughter's dieting behaviors, she recounted similar weight-loss strategies, eating patterns, and food choices. However, she also identified a critical difference: each generation within her family started dieting at a significantly younger age. The majority of mothers I have counseled and interviewed describe the same pattern. They realize that they have followed in their mothers' dieting footsteps and that their daughters are following in theirs—but at a much accelerated pace.

To help you gain an understanding of the generational transfer of unhealthy weight-loss behaviors, reflect on your own family by comparing your mother's, yours, and your daughter's dieting practices—the ages you started, the methods you used, and the effect that dieting has had on your lives.

Do You Remember
Your Mother Dieting?

You may have memories similar to one of my clients who vividly recalled the day her mother started dieting. "I was eleven years old when she and her friends were in the kitchen looking at pictures of Twiggy and reading through *Dr. Atkin's Diet Revolution.* I think she spent most of her thirties eating the typical diet plate of a bunless hamburger patty and side of cottage cheese. Thirty years later she still skimps on carbohydrates and anxiously awaits the next 'guaranteed' weight-loss gimmick."

Most of our mothers began dieting in the 1960s and '70s. Eager to imitate the models of the day, they jumped on the dieting bandwagon and became the disciples of the low-carbohydrate, high-protein diets. For our mothers' generation, dieting was an exciting new trend that offered an alternative female identity, a freedom from the traditional matronly image of their mothers. This trend caught on quickly as more women's magazines hit the market and as television viewing became the most popular form of entertainment. For the first time in history, millions could simultaneously view anorexic-looking models on the news and on the newsstand. At about the same time, the first medical reports on the health hazards of obesity were also making headlines, the Metropolitan Life Insurance Company introduced its height/weight charts recommending lower weights, and doctors began urging weight loss. The convergence of a new, thin female identity, the medical warnings of obesity, and the increased influence of the media all made dieting an overnight trend and weight loss a primary goal.

Unaware how deeply this new trend would affect them, trap their daughters, and imprison their granddaughters, our mothers gave birth to a new culture of dieting. And we, their daughters, were the first generation to be raised by calorie-counting mothers who were preoccupied with their weight and forever dependent on the bathroom scale for evaluation of their self-worth.

How Do Your Dieting Behaviors Compare to Your Mother's?

One client answered, "My mother put me on my first diet at age fourteen, and I've barely come up for air since. But I'm much more serious about dieting than my mother ever was. A day doesn't go by that I don't think about the calories in food and the pounds on my body."

Our mothers may have been the first to experiment with fad dieting, but my generation (and I expect yours too) began dieting as teenagers and declared it our lifelong career. We made the 1980s' diet books—from *The Beverly Hills Diet,* which advocated the use of raw fruit to induce diarrhea (in reality a form of bulimia), to *Dr. Berger's Immune Power Diet,* which eliminated all milk, wheat, eggs, and sugar—guaranteed best-sellers. We also lined up at the booming new weight-loss centers and sampled all their programs, from Weight Watchers, to Diet Center, to Nutrisystem, to Jenny Craig, to Optifast—and then back to Weight Watchers again to re-peat the cycle. Our mothers joined these programs too, but we were the ones who became repeat customers. The diet industry has us to thank for making it the $30 billion business it is today.[5] Unfortu-nately, the only thank-you gift we've gotten is thicker fat pads for our thighs because our repeated dieting efforts have only left us fatter. The average woman has lost about 100 pounds by dieting, only to regain 125.

Our weight losses and gains are due not only to the many tra-ditional diet plans and programs we've tried and failed but also to a variety of "new" forms of dieting: we're now counting grams of fat, cutting out sugar, giving up our favorite foods, eliminating red meat, and eating primarily fruits and vegetables. We may think that we're following a healthy eating plan or a lifestyle program, but if the purpose is quick weight loss, then we're really following a diet.

We are also the first generation to practice another type of dieting you probably haven't heard of before—*unnecessary dieting.* Now, in my opinion, all dieting is unnecessary, but it's especially unnecessary for those who are at a healthy weight and have never been overweight by health standards. Most of our mothers dieted because they were medically overweight; many of us are dieting not because we are overweight but because we *feel* overweight.

We gaze in the mirror and ask the proverbial question: "Mirror, mirror on the wall, who's the skinniest of them all?" As we grab at our thighs, we answer before the magical mirror has a chance: "Not you; look at that fat on the back of your thighs and those love handles on your hips. Half of your friends are thinner than you are. Better lose some more weight—starting today."

If we had allowed the mirror to assess our body size accurately, most of us would be reassured. Some hip and thigh fat is not only healthy, it's essential for menstruation and fertility. But distorted body images, weight misperceptions, and unrealistic and unhealthy weight expectations have resulted in a new population of female dieters who are of normal and below-normal weight. Studies show that over one-half of all women dieting today are *not* overweight.

Our mothers started the dieting trend, and we have followed them eagerly, with even greater determination. Now many of us have daughters of our own, and they are already aware that they are daughters of dieting mothers: 69 percent of the adolescent girls surveyed report that their mothers diet, but only 13 percent describe their mothers as overweight.[6] What does this say to our young daughters? That dieting is normal behavior for normal-weight women? That appears to be the message given and, as a result, playing grown-up has taken on a sinister new meaning.

HOW DO YOUR DAUGHTER'S DIETING BEHAVIORS COMPARE TO YOURS?

A concerned mother responded, "My daughter started talking about her weight when she was eight years old. Now, at age eleven, she gets on the scale every morning, seldom eats breakfast or lunch, and recently informed me that she was becoming a no-fat vegetarian. I'm worried about her and her friends; they shouldn't be obsessing about their weight at their age."

I share this mother's concern. Young girls today are in a dieting category all their own. They have accepted the slender ideal, measured themselves against it, and have decided that even in a prepubescent state, they come up fat. The following research summary will alert you to the alarming chronology of our dieting daughters:

- By age five, they describe thin friends as being more desirable than overweight friends.[7]
- By age six, they have internalized the slender ideal, and 40 percent have expressed a desire to be thinner.[8]
- By age nine, their desire has translated into action, and nearly 50 percent have already embarked on their first restrictive diet.[9]
- By age ten, more than half voice their fear of becoming fat.[10]
- By age thirteen, 80 percent of the adolescent girls are dieting to fight the natural changes in their maturing bodies.[11]
- By age fifteen, one out of eight teenage girls is dieting at least ten times a year.[12]
- By age sixteen, 45 percent are crash dieting, 40 percent are fasting, and 15 percent are taking diet pills.[13]
- By age seventeen, four out of five healthy-weight young women think they are too fat.[14]
- By age twenty, 95 percent express a strong desire to lose weight.[15]

If these young women don't stop dieting, virtually all of the third generation, our future female leaders, will be consumed with weight worries, spending half of their adult lives trying to lose weight and the other half gaining it back. They will also likely be plagued with health problems. The damage report from dieting is lengthy and includes menstrual irregularities, thyroid problems, fatigue, hair loss, and bone loss, to mention only some of the consequences. Our daughters are dieting their way to hormonal dysfunction and body dissatisfaction.

If they are worrying about their thighs at age nine, how will they function at age twenty-nine? If they have been on ten diets by age fifteen, how much of their lives will they waste dieting by age forty-five? *If they feel fat at age six, how are they going to feel about their bodies as mature women?*

How old were you when you first "felt fat"? I know that I was closer to sixteen than six. I remember sitting in my high school cafeteria when, all of a sudden, I was overwhelmed with a feeling of fatness. When we say that we "feel fat," we are really saying that we're not feeling good about ourselves; we're feeling self-conscious, inadequate, or uncomfortable. I know now that when I had that "fat flash" as a sixteen-year-old, I was not at all fat, but my state of mind triggered dieting as a way to feel confident and in control by being thin.

"Feeling fat" is a new, accepted, and widely used entry in our and our daughters' emotional vocabulary. Even before young daughters are able to identify the full spectrum of their feelings, they seem to know what it means to "feel fat." I'd like to underscore the emergence of this phenomenon by recounting recent interviews with two normal-weight young girls: the first, a six-year-old, told me that she doesn't like wearing a bathing suit because she "feels" too fat, and the other, a nine-year-old, revealed that she sometimes stays home from school because she "feels" fat.

The dieting trend is *not* diminishing; instead it's accelerating. With each of the past three generations of women, the daughters of dieters start dieting younger, diet more, and have poorer body images. *Younger and younger girls are being initiated into the dangerous world of dieting, and many are surpassing the previous generation by the time they reach adolescence.*

Have you discovered that your mother, you, and/or your daughter are caught in the trap of dieting?

An estimated 70 percent of you will answer "yes" to this question. If you did, then you may be asking some questions of your own: Why didn't anyone inform you that the dieting epidemic was reaching your daughter? Why weren't you aware that your dieting practices would be passed on to your daughter? Why weren't you more prepared to help your daughter avoid the dieting trap?

How could you have been informed, aware, or prepared? Because weight preoccupation and body dissatisfaction have become a part of the indoctrination into womanhood, little advice has been given on this unspoken childhood calamity. Dieting is firmly in-

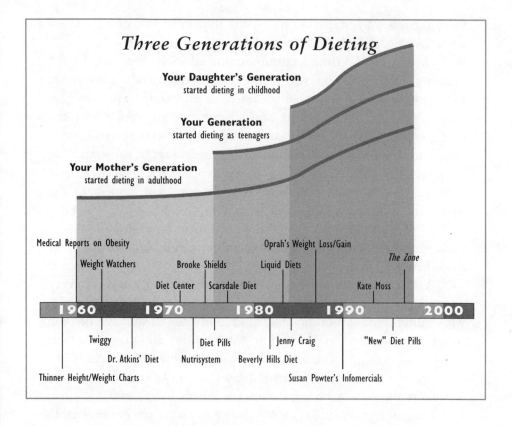

grained in our society because what began as a trend almost forty years ago is now a culture.

THE CULTURE OF DIETING

Of course my daughter and I diet. Don't all women?
—Penny, age 39

Fashions change, music changes, technology changes—but dieting doesn't. Dieting has withstood the test of time. Every fad, pop culture, and subgroup values the thin ideal and advocates the practice of dieting. From the yuppies to Generation X, from rock and roll to rap, from polyester to grunge—the thin image prevails and dictates the ideal female body.

Dieting has become a culture in and of itself. Practiced by the majority, dieting has its own identifiable system of ideas, methods, values, beliefs, and norms that constrain and shape our thoughts and actions. At times, dieting and weight loss are even a national event. Oprah's weight loss*es* (and weight gains) have received more media coverage than other newsworthy world events; the search for an antidote to the obesity gene is headline news; and a recent *People Magazine* cover story boasted "Diet Winners and Sinners of the Year: The Skinny on Who Got Fat, Who Got Fit, and How They Did It." Celebrities now shrink and expand in front of 280 million people, and our daughters watch them on television and form their own dieting value system.

As for the rules and regulations of dieting—I could fill every page of this book with the "can't haves" and "don'ts" associated with eating. Eating morality and food fundamentalism have become so universal that we are judged at home, work, and play, and then we serve as self-appointed judges in our daughters' food court. As mothers, we preside over the food laws of the land and teach our daughters that less is best and thinness breeds happiness.

For prior generations, most eating rules were reserved for table manners. The main "don'ts" were don't eat with your hands and don't put your elbows on the table. Other eating rules were reserved for those with health conditions. For diabetics, the rule was don't eat sugar; for those with a wheat allergy, it was don't eat wheat; for those with gallbladder disease, it was don't eat fat. Otherwise, "eat, drink, and be merry," as the saying goes.

Today's motto is closer to **"don't eat, don't drink, or be sorry."**

To further add to dieting's cultural significance, dieting has developed a quasi-language of its own. One young client called it "diet speak," and it has given many words an entirely different meaning, including the word "diet." The following are some examples of current and former usage:

- **diet**—now means a reduction in calories to promote weight loss instead of one's overall daily food intake

- **purging**—now means vomiting food instead of ridding the body of a harmful, undesirable substance, such as poison
- **burn**—now means utilizing calories or body fat to produce heat instead of igniting wood
- **skipping**—now refers to missing a meal instead of a pace
- **yo-yo**—now describes repeated dieting instead of a bobbing toy
- **junk**—now describes a type of food instead of useless waste

Despite its identifiable values, beliefs, rules, and language, the culture of dieting defies sociological theory. Cultures are supposed to evolve to allow society to function efficiently and orderly. Without them, we would rely on raw, biological instincts that would eventually cause chaos. Our biological eating instincts, however, would serve us much better for efficient functioning than does the culture of dieting. Dieting has created mass eating and weight chaos: little girls dieting; underweight women undereating; women dying from self-starvation; women isolating themselves from society with self-induced vomiting; women fasting and abusing laxatives, diuretics, and diet pills. These unhealthy, maladaptive weight-loss behaviors are caused by dieting and are the legacy that's being endowed to our daughters.

THE LEGACY OF DISORDERED EATING

Oh, my daughter doesn't have an eating problem. She takes diet pills and exercises a lot, but she doesn't vomit, so you don't have to be worried about her.
—Belinda, age 45

Despite this admonition, I was extremely worried about Belinda's teenage daughter. She was running forty miles a week, hooked on diet pills, and eating only 800 calories a day. Every day she would ask herself, "How can I eat less and burn up the food that I do eat before it's lodged in my thighs?"

She is joined by millions of other women, young and old, who ask the same or similar questions. "How can I lose a pound today?" or "How can I eat less today?" or "How can I burn up some fat today?" The only possible answer is through drastic weight-loss attempts that border on eating disorders. I call them *disordered eating behaviors.* At one extreme are the eating disorders, anorexia and bulimia, and many mothers feel that if their daughters aren't hospitalized for self-starvation or self-induced vomiting, then they don't have an eating problem. But they still may have a severe eating problem because they are on the verge of becoming eating disorder victims.

Any woman who has some form of an unhealthy relationship with food and her body is a disordered eater. She may be caught in the diet/binge cycle, restricting "forbidden" foods, feeling guilty after eating, or in a semistarvation state from chronic undereating, fasting, skipping meals, or overexercising. This may very well be you, your daughter, your mother, and many of your friends.

Are you beginning to wonder if you and/or your daughter have a form of disordered eating?

One frivolous diet attempt does not lead to disordered eating, but do you know of any woman who has dieted once, then stopped forever? I don't. Once you start dieting, you're usually hooked. You diet, lose some weight, gain the weight back, then diet harder and gain the weight back quicker. Then diet even harder . . . and so on.

Three important questions can help you determine whether you and/or your daughter is a disordered eater:

- Do you and/or your daughter fear weight gain?
- Do you and/or your daughter think about what you weigh and what you will and will not allow yourself to eat on a daily basis?
- Do you and/or your daughter practice any of the following weight-loss attempts: on again–off again dieting, skipping meals, twenty-four-hour fasts, diet pills, excessive exercise, diuretics, laxatives, or vomiting?

From the various national surveys, an estimated 60 percent of adult women and perhaps as much as 80 percent of teenage girls can be categorized as disordered eaters. They fear weight gain, are preoccupied with their weight and food intake, and are constantly figuring out a way to rid their bodies of weight and food.

These drastic, unhealthy weight-loss attempts have become increasingly characteristic of our daughters' generation. The National Adolescent Healthy Survey found that 51 percent had fasted, 16 percent had taken diet pills, and 12 percent had vomited in the last month.[16] In another analysis of tenth-grade dieting females, more than 65 percent admitted to using unhealthy, dangerous methods such as prolonged fasting, diet pills, laxatives, and vomiting.[17]

In fact, they do more than admit to these unhealthy weight-loss methods. They discuss dieting, purging, and fasting quite nonchalantly. When I asked one seventh grader about her weight control practices, she answered matter-of-factly, "I make sure I stay a little hungry all day long, and I sometimes take laxatives when I think I'm getting fat, but I have a friend who takes laxatives, runs ten miles, and throws up every day. I wish I could make myself throw up so that I could be as thin as she is." Some adult women have told me at least half jokingly that they wish they would "get" anorexia, but this thirteen-year-old was dead serious.

From my observations, this new generation of young daughters views disordered eating as an acceptable, even desirable practice. I have been counseling dieters, anorexics, bulimics, and compulsive overeaters for fifteen years, and I know that adult women are much more secretive about their eating behaviors. They are aware of the harm they are doing to their bodies with fasting, bingeing, and purging, and they often go to many extremes to keep these unhealthy behaviors a secret from family and friends. But today's female youth doesn't feel the need to hide them. Disordered eating practices have become so commonplace that one fourteen-year-old told me that it was "totally uncool to eat lunch" and that "you had to be obsessed with weight loss to fit in."

The cultural reaction to the increase in female dieting practices, disordered eating behaviors, and even eating disorders has been akin to "Well, girls will be girls." Fear of fat, dieting, weight preoccupation, negative body image, and other disordered eating behaviors are considered normal passages of womanhood. But is it normal to avoid a social function because we feel fat? Is it normal for our daughters to diet their way to disordered eating? Is it normal for women of any age to put their lives on hold until they are thin?

When we spend a moment thinking about these questions, our firm response is "NO!" It's not normal to wake up every day unhappy about our weight and uncomfortable with our bodies. Just because the majority of all women share these disordered eating patterns doesn't make them normal—*it makes them endemic.*

As many as 8 million American women and girls have eating disorders, 80 million have dieted, and 100 million "feel fat" regardless of their weight. These figures describe the unhealthy, abnormal legacy of disordered eating that has already trapped two generations of women and is quickly being absorbed by a third. At the same time, another epidemic is parallelling this one: *obesity.* Many of us and our daughters are not only disordered eaters, we're *overweight disordered eaters.*

THE EPIDEMIC OF OBESITY

The more diets I've been on, the fatter I've become. I'm an overweight dieter and my daughter is too.
—Barbara, age 47

It may seem both paradoxical and confusing that a rise in obesity is occurring at the same time as an increase in dieting and disordered eating. But many dieters are overweight because dieting can cause both disordered eating *and* obesity.

Obesity is defined as being more than 20 percent over your recommended healthy weight. This definition surprises many women who thought obesity meant being at least 100 pounds overweight. As you can see, much overlap exists between the terms "overweight" and "obese," and often they are used interchangeably. But the incidence of both *overweight* and *obesity* is on the rise.

The last decade has produced the biggest jump in obesity in

history. For adult women, obesity increased by 36 percent and now includes more than one out of every three women.[18] And for the six- to eleven-year-olds, the increase has topped 50 percent![19]

Although some women's family history biases them toward obesity, the rise cannot be explained by genetics. It's impossible for our genes to have mutated in one decade, but it's entirely possible for our yo-yo dieting habits to have changed individual body chemistries over the last ten years to cause this kind of weight gain across the female population.

More mothers are dieting; more daughters are dieting. More mothers are disordered eaters; more daughters are disordered eaters. More mothers are overweight; more daughters are overweight. This sequence is not coincidental. *Dieting is the primary cause of all our weight and eating problems.*

Now, some women are disordered eaters because a traumatic event in their lives, such as physical abuse or rape, has triggered their unhealthy eating behavior as a defense mechanism. Other women are overweight because they are genetically prone or because they haven't stopped eating long enough to consider dieting. But for most women, the number-one factor preceding disordered eating and obesity *is* dieting—and the long-debated "chicken or the egg" question can now be answered.

Are more women dieting because more women are overweight?

or

Are more women overweight because more women are dieting?

More women are overweight because more women are dieting. Dieting leads to weight gain in one of two ways.

First, we undereat while we're on the diet. Undereating undermines our metabolism, or ability to burn calories, so that we gain weight on fewer calories. The typical woman eats about 200 calories *less* and weighs about eight pounds *more* than she did thirty years ago when she first started dieting.

Second, we overeat when we come off the diet. What do you do to celebrate the finale of your six-week diet? Go out for a six-course dinner? When all willpower reserves are gone, what happens to your diet? You get the point. Dieting causes overindulgence.

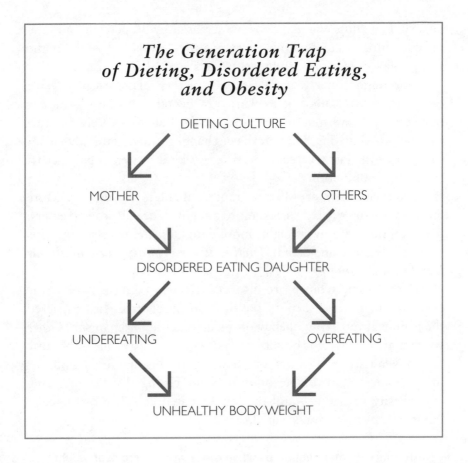

*The Generation Trap
of Dieting, Disordered Eating,
and Obesity*

DIETING CULTURE

MOTHER   OTHERS

DISORDERED EATING DAUGHTER

UNDEREATING   OVEREATING

UNHEALTHY BODY WEIGHT

First we undereat and slow down our metabolism when we're on the diet, then we overeat and quickly gain weight when we go off the diet.

If you are overweight, it's most likely because you are dieting or have had a long history of dieting—and a sedentary lifestyle (more on that later). If you have a daughter, her chances for obesity will be increased if you encourage her to diet. You may be causing the very condition that you seek to prevent.

Although mothers are the most influential in passing on the legacy of disordered eating and obesity, they are not the only ones who help to ensure its passage. Sisters, grandmothers, aunts, fathers, husbands, boyfriends, peers, fashion models, celebrities, and mentors have all been influenced by society's thin ideal and the culture of dieting—and they all help to keep our daughters caught in the generation trap of dieting, disordered eating, and obesity.

Society's thin ideal and the culture of dieting may be responsible for the existence of this trap, but our own dieting behaviors and negative attitudes keep us and our daughters helplessly stuck. Therefore, by taking charge of our own relationship with food, *we possess the key to setting ourselves and our daughters free.*

BREAKING FREE FROM THE GENERATION TRAP

> *If dieting causes eating problems and obesity, then why do we choose to do it?*
>
> —*Kirin, age 9*

This astute young daughter asked the million-dollar question. Dieting is a choice. We are not being forced to diet, we do so because we are being strongly persuaded by the values, beliefs, and norms within our culture. But, for our own well-being and especially for our daughters', we can make an intelligent, well-informed choice *not* to diet.

And instead, we can choose to raise our daughters in a diet-free environment, teach them to listen to their bodies' needs, and listen to our own bodies' needs. And, if enough women make these choices for themselves and their daughters, the generation trap of disordered eating can be transformed into a women's liberation of healthy food and body relationships.

I often wonder what, hundreds of years from now, anthropologists, sociologists, and historians will conclude about this disordered eating phenomenon. That we needed to shrink our bodies to take up less space because of overpopulation? That we worshipped the skin-and-bones look? That we were purposely weakened by dieting? That we purposely weakened ourselves because of our ambivalence about entering a man's world (as some antifeminists propose)? That we subconsciously molded our bodies into a tubelike shape because of penis envy (as some Freudians may believe)?

I certainly don't want to be remembered that way. I want to be known as a proud member of the three generations of women who joined together to help themselves and each other break free from the generation trap to ensure a healthy eating legacy for their daughters and future generations of women.

As a nutritionist dedicated to women's health and as a woman concerned about the future of our gender, I encourage you to take part in creating the necessary counterculture of anti-dieting and the formation of healthier eating legacies. It must start in your own home by breaking the pattern of disordered eating and transforming your mother/daughter food and body relationship to a more positive one. To do so, first you must recognize the many different ways you may be influencing the eating habits and body image of the daughter you love.

CHAPTER TWO

MOTHERS
UNKNOWINGLY
PASSING THE TORCH

A *mother called me* up one morning concerned about her eleven-year-old daughter who was bingeing on "junk" food and rapidly gaining weight. As she was describing her daughter's eating behavior, I asked about her own eating habits, and she replied, "I'm so careful about what I eat; I can't believe that she doesn't care. I have a very low-fat diet, and I never eat sugar, snack, or allow junk food in the house. But I'm finding empty potato chip bags and candy wrappers everywhere. I've done everything I can to make sure my daughter eats right. I've put her on a low-fat diet, forbidden snacking, and set up a reward system for her to lose weight. I don't understand why she is eating junk and putting on weight."

After explaining to this mother how restriction, control, and eating rules inevitably backfire, she fully understood why her daughter was rebelling and going against her well-intentioned wishes. You too will come to understand how your good food intentions can have unexpected outcomes and how your own relationship with food can negatively affect your daughter's. For example, if you:

- enforce strict eating rules
- restrict your daughter's fat and sugar intake
- restrict your own fat and sugar intake
- exercise control over your daughter's eating habits
- encourage your daughter to diet
- diet
- weigh yourself and feel uncomfortable with your body

then you are in some way passing the torch of dieting, disordered eating, and body dissatisfaction on to your daughter. If your mother practiced any of these behaviors, then she passed the legacy on to you. Please don't let this cause any anxiety now. I will help you to understand the reasons behind your mother's actions with you and your actions with your daughter. While at times this learning process may be painful, it will also be insightful and motivating. In order to gain the confidence and skills to reverse the disordered eating trend, first you have to know what you are doing to reinforce it with your daughter. *Rest assured, virtually all mothers who are passing the unhealthy legacy are doing so unknowingly.*

Based on society's eating rules as well as on recent findings from nutrition and medical research, you are doing what you think is best for your daughter's health and well-being. You may have heard that arterial plaque formation begins at age three, that a growing number of children have high blood pressure and high blood cholesterol levels, that cancer risk starts in childhood, and that extra body fat increases the risk of almost every disease and decreases the chances of academic, career, and marital success.

What's a mother to do?

We care about our daughters and want to be good mothers, so we quickly take on the responsibility of revamping their eating habits by removing excess fat, sugar, salt, cholesterol, and calories from their diets. We may be doing what we think is best, but what we don't know is that our underlying good intentions can have long-lasting consequences.

MOTHER'S GOOD FOOD INTENTIONS

*I'm doing everything I can to make sure that my daughter
is eating right. I never have junk food in the house and
have never once brought her to McDonald's.*

—Mary, age 42

What exactly is the definition of eating right? These days, eating right usually means eating *less*:

- eating *less* fat
- eating *less* cholesterol
- eating *less* sugar
- eating *less* salt
- eating *less* red meat
- eating *less* processed foods
- eating *less* junk food
- eating *fewer* snacks

We are led to believe that if we make sure our daughters abide by these socially accepted eating rules, they will be healthy and lean. First of all, however, there is no guarantee that these goals will be reached. Diet is but one of the many risk factors for disease and only one of the many variables that affect weight. Second, a restrictive eating approach will almost surely backfire by bringing about disordered eating and/or obesity. And third, feelings of deprivation and guilt will eventually set in. When your daughter does eat "forbidden" high-fat and -sugar foods, she'll overeat them and then feel guilty. In fact, over 50 percent of our adolescent daughters surveyed report that they feel guilty after overeating.[1]

You didn't make up these limiting eating rules; rather they reflect a restrictive dieting culture, one endorsed by many physicians, nutritionists, aerobics instructors, personal trainers, friends, family members, newspaper journalists, magazine editors, teachers, and coaches. You are simply serving as society's messenger and passing along the ever growing bundle of food negativism and nutrition misinformation to your daughter.

As part of the research for this book, I surveyed over 100 mothers in the San Francisco Bay Area on what their priorities were when feeding their preadolescent daughters. Here are their top five answers as well as examples of how good food intentions can ultimately lead to unhealthy eating behaviors.

1. **Limit junk food in my daughter's diet** was the number-one response. Some mothers reported keeping no chips or cookies in the house; others allowed "junk" food only for special treats or practiced the one-junk-food-a-day philosophy. Their good intentions are obvious; they wanted to ensure a higher nutritional quality in their daughters' diets and a lower intake of fat, sugar, salt, and preservatives. When I asked how well this food strategy was working, most were less than pleased. They found cookies hidden under their daughters' beds or discovered that their daughters were vacuuming out the junk food cupboard at friends' homes. One mother discovered that her daughter was spending her entire allowance at the candy counter, while another was unaware that her daughter had become the local Burger King's most popular customer—until I shared the news. Children are no different from adults. It's human nature to always want what you can't have. And, with food, your daughter may go to extremes to get it.

2. **Put her on a low-fat diet** has replaced "put her on a low-calorie diet," but reducing fat is usually just another way to reduce calories. One of the primary motives may be to prevent heart disease fifty years from now, but when you cut out fat, you cut out calories as well as much of the taste and satisfaction. One mother was quite proud of her educational efforts; she was teaching her daughter how to count by adding up the grams of fat she was eating each day. Whatever happened to counting marbles or pennies? Other mothers are now stocking their kitchen with anything that says "nonfat" on it: nonfat cookies, nonfat crackers, nonfat hot dogs, nonfat cheese, and nonfat chips. Young girls are learn-

ing that nonfat is good, fat is bad, and if you eat anything but a "nonfat" food, you are a bad person.

3. **No sweets in the house** to promote dental health and prevent obesity is considered a healthy child-feeding practice. One mother who had no sweets in the house for over ten years knew she had made a mistake when her daughter recently moved into an apartment and immediately filled her cupboards and refrigerator with anything and everything high in sugar just because "she could." Other mothers only allowed whole-grain cereals with no added sugar. These mothers reported that it was difficult to get their young daughters to eat breakfast because they were forever pleading to go "coo-coo over Cocoa Puffs" or get a cereal that contained a hidden prize. To tell you the truth, I have a difficult time getting excited about turbo-fiber cereals that taste like shredded twigs held together with cardboard paste. Children have a greater number of sugar taste buds on the tip of their tongue that increase their preference for sugar. If they are unsatisfied at breakfast or any other meal, they will try to make up for it later with more sugar.

4. **No snacking between meals** is another common family food rule, and mothers continue to believe that three balanced meals a day provide the best nutrition and prevent excess calories. But the reality is that children (and most women too) get hungry every three to four hours because their bodies and brains need a constant source of fuel. Snacking provides nutrients and contributes significantly to their iron, magnesium, and B vitamin intake.[2] Depriving them of snacks may deprive them of nutrients and make them irritable, lethargic, overhungry—and encourage them to overeat at meals.

5. **Make sure that she cleans her plate** was the only priority that pushed food intake rather than restricted it. From my own experience and from the research findings, most mothers are restricting their daughters' eating, yet enough mothers are enforcing plate cleaning to make it one of the top five priorities. Most of us were brought up with the dinnertime clean-your-plate creed, and we're still having a difficult time leaving a morsel of food

behind. One adult daughter describes herself as a "human garbage disposal" because she cleans her plate first, then cleans everyone else's plates before she puts them in the dishwasher. Another adult daughter with nightmarish memories of cleaning her plate of macaroni and cheese can't bring herself to eat the dish thirty years later. Haven't we learned that lesson? We know what the clean-your-plate rule has done to us, yet some of us continue to use the same bribes, threats, and rewards on our daughters:

> "If you don't finish what's on your plate, you'll go to bed early."

> "You'll sit there until your plate is clean, even if you have to sit there all night."

> "Finish your peas, and you'll get ice cream for dessert."

Not only do these techniques not work very well, they can have deleterious effects. For example, forced pea consumption with the reward of ice cream has been found to decrease the preference for peas and increase the preference for ice cream.[3] Whoops! If you want your daughter to eat her peas, you should be doing the opposite and using peas as the reward. Can you imagine yourself saying "Finish your ice cream, and you can have some peas"?

Whether it's with forced plate cleaning or restrictive feeding, trying to control your daughter's food intake will inevitably backfire.

CONTROL *IS* COUNTERPRODUCTIVE

My mother acts like she's captain of the food police. She monitors everything I eat and puts me on the scale every day.

—Ashley, age 17

Ashley has a younger sister, Amy, and the two siblings have had opposite reactions to their mother's "food policing." Ashley has rebelled against her mother by eating everything she can get her hands on as soon as she is out of the house while Amy has become her mother's protégé, welcoming the control and internalizing the food restrictive behavior as her own. Restrictive feeding can cause either side of disordered eating.

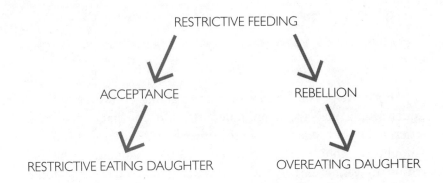

If you restrict your daughter's food intake, she will react in one of two ways by either:

rebelling—"No way!"—and overeating when you're not looking

or

accepting—"Okay!"—and not eating at all when you're not looking.

She'll be eating when she's not hungry, or she'll be denying her body food when she is hungry. Whichever her reaction, you have taught her not to trust her body's internal food messages.

The same is true if you attempt to overfeed your daughter. She may rebel and avoid food when she's out of the house. Or she will consider overeating normal, acceptable behavior and continue to do so when she's away from home and years later when she has a home of her own. You are teaching her to eat more than she needs and teaching her body to store the excess calories as fat. Again, you are telling your daughter not to trust her body's food messages.

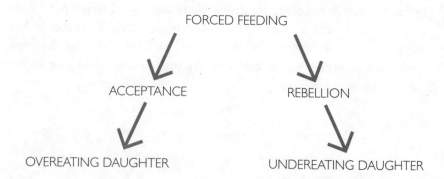

It's quite possible that mothers are giving both overfeeding and underfeeding messages simultaneously. On one hand, they are restricting fat and sugar. But on the other hand, they are pushing large amounts of nonfat foods to make sure their daughters' diet is nutritionally balanced. Daughters are getting mixed messages: don't eat fat so you won't become fat, but eat a lot of nonfat foods that will become fat anyway. Fat is the storage form of all excess calories. Even if we only overfeed our daughters rice cakes, that food too will be converted to fat and stored as fat.

Social and cognitive research on parenting style and childhood development has shown that a controlling parenting style hinders the child's ability to develop internal self-control.[4] This is true in all areas of behavior, including food and weight. Understanding these findings can help any mother concerned about her daughter's eating habits and body weight.

If you exert external control and decide when, what, and how much your daughter will eat, she will lose touch with her body's internal control mechanisms. This consequence is unfortunate because listening to the body's internal food needs and responding to physiological hunger and fullness cues are keys to healthy eating *and* permanent weight control. Your daughter is the expert in defining the whats, whys, and whens of her eating—not you and not society's eating rules. This is true from infancy through adulthood.

One of my favorite infant studies used different concentrations of formula. When the formula was diluted, the infants drank more, and when the formula was more concentrated, they drank less— each time perfectly adjusting the amount themselves so that they consumed about the same number of calories.[5] Studies on older children and adolescents have shown the same results: children *can* regulate their own food intake appropriately; they don't need to be restrained or pushed—and when they are, they get confused, no longer knowing whether to listen to their bodies or to their mothers. And this confusion has a lasting effect. College students who were fed restrictively in childhood continued to restrict their own food intake in adulthood—and were also more likely to be overweight.[6]

But most mothers are not aware of the counterproductive effects of food control and become more frustrated as their daughters' weight begins to climb. Their increased anxieties cause them to exercise even more control and to begin control at ever younger ages. One study investigating underweight one-year-old daughters who were referred to a pediatrician for poor weight gain found that the majority of the mothers thought their daughters to be of normal weight (when in fact they were extremely underweight, at the third percentile or below) and were purposefully restricting sweets and other "fattening" foods to prevent weight gain.[7]

Another extreme example is of a mother I know who stopped breast-feeding her daughter when she heard that breast milk was high in fat. She weaned her infant straight to nonfat milk, and the result was devastating: her one-year-old daughter was admitted to the hospital for essential fatty acid deficiency and failure to thrive. This woman's behavior indicates the urgent need to educate mothers on the vital nutritional needs of infants and children, and the life-threatening result when they aren't met. All infants and children need fat in their diets to prevent deficiencies and to provide the necessary calories for healthy growth. And severe restriction during infancy and childhood can overstimulate the appetite center and guarantee an overweight daughter later in life. *At every stage of development, restrictive feeding does not "save" the daughter from an overweight fate, it ensures it.*

Now, if you also have a son, do you feed him differently? Most mothers do. Some researchers have documented that infant sons receive, on average, 50 percent more breast-feeding time than daughters.[8] And as infant sons mature into young boys, mothers are less likely to control their food intake and more likely to trust their internal eating cues.[9] Mothers do not serve as the primary role models for sons, nor do they project their own weight dreams onto their sons as they do with their daughters.

Let me pause here to talk about internal control and external control. Studies use these technical terms, but we don't use them conversationally. *Internal control* means that eating habits are guided by the body's instinctive physiological hunger and fullness signals. *External control* means that our eating habits are guided by willpower, discipline, guilt, emotions, society's eating rules, diet plans, the clock, and other environmental cues. From now on, I'd like to use less clinical but more descriptive phrases: *instinctive eating* instead of internal control and *disordered eating* (I've been using this one all along) instead of external control. Too much external control overrides instinctive eating and causes disordered eating. How would you describe your eating behavior? Are you a disordered eater or an instinctive eater?

If you are a disordered eater

- you are more likely to try to control your daughter's eating
- your daughter is more likely to become a disordered eater
- your daughter is more likely to be overweight
- you are more likely to be overweight

But if you are an instinctive eater

- you are more likely to trust your daughter's eating decisions
- your daughter is more likely to become an instinctive eater
- your daughter is more likely to maintain a comfortable weight
- you are more likely to maintain a comfortable weight

We are all born with instincts that direct us to eat when we need fuel and to stop eating when we have consumed an adequate amount. But if you don't respect your own eating signals, you are teaching your daughter that she shouldn't respect hers. If you control your daughter's eating, you are severing her instinctive eating mechanisms and destroying her ability to maintain a healthy weight.

Of course, the solution is to stop controlling our daughters' eating habits and start trusting their eating instincts. This is difficult for many mothers because they are out of touch with their own eating instincts, struggling to control their own eating habits, and failing at the weight-loss game. Are you one of these women?

Family systems research has shown that mothers are most controlling in the areas in which they are personally invested.[10] Well, the typical adult woman feels out of control with her own eating habits, goes on at least fifteen diets in her lifetime, and spends a portion of the annual family income on weight loss. No one would argue that most mothers are highly invested in dieting and disordered eating. Because they perceive themselves as unable to control their own food intake and weight, they believe that their daughters are also incapable of self-control and consequently take on the responsibility of controlling what, when, and how much the daughters eat.

Research has also shown that mothers who view their daughters as extensions of themselves are more controlling in the areas in which they perceive themselves as having failed. Almost all women have failed in their attempts to achieve the perfect body. Our unrealistic expectations ensure failure, as do our methods. With a documented failure rate of 98 percent,[11] dieting is a no-win situation. As one mother said, "I've tried, failed, and I'll be damned if my daughter fails too."

Unfortunately, it's your daughter who will be damned. The more food control you impose and the more you encourage her to diet, the less food control your daughter will have—and the more she will struggle with her weight in the years to come.

DO YOU ENCOURAGE YOUR DAUGHTER TO DIET?

I diet with my daughter to give her moral support.
—Sophia, age 38

Do you think your daughter needs to lose weight? If so, how much weight do you think she needs to lose? Twenty pounds, ten pounds, five pounds? One study asked this very same question, and regardless of their daughters' weight, mothers who were disordered eaters wanted their daughters to lose an average of twelve pounds whereas mothers who were not disordered eaters thought their daughters should stay right where they were.[12]

What are you doing, if anything, to encourage your daughter to diet?

Dieting with her is, of course, the most direct method of encouragement, and from my experience, it happens all too frequently. Karen calls herself and her daughter "codependent dieters" because they have been dieting together for over twenty-five years. "When one of us decides it's time to go on another diet, then the other one is there by her side. And when one of us decides it's time to go off the diet, the other one says 'The hell with it' too." This mother/daughter dieting team had a great sense of humor and were more lighthearted in their approach to dieting than most. They used to laugh all the way to the weight-loss clinic as they were reminiscing about their last diet and laugh all the way home as they were sneaking a package of cookies in the car. They made me laugh when they shared one of their most ridiculous weight-loss attempts. Last year they decided to go "cold turkey" to give up chocolate, and that's literally all they ate for two weeks—cold turkey breast.

I wish we all had such a good sense of dieting humor, but most of us take the dieting game much more seriously. When Stephanie and her daughter dieted, it meant no socializing, no restaurants, and no fun. Each night they reviewed each other's food records by adding up the calories and grams of fat. They had a system of grading each other, and if they got below a B−, they were put in detention the next day and were allowed only 500 calories.

Whether it's with laughter or loneliness, if you and your daughter are dietmates, then you are directly teaching her that dieting is the ultimate control strategy and a necessary female ritual that must be repeated many, many times throughout a woman's life. If you support her dieting attempts by buying all nonfat foods, preparing special meals, or weighing her, then you are teaching her that dieting is acceptable, normal behavior.

And what if your daughter is overweight? Hundreds of mothers of overweight daughters have asked me, "Should I put her on a diet?

Should I restrict her calorie, fat, and sugar intake?" Absolutely not!! Dieting will only make her preoccupied with food and cause more fat storage. Furthermore, the vast majority of overweight daughters are *not* overeating. Most studies have shown that heavier children are already eating less than leaner children. (Needless to say, they are also exercising less than leaner children—more on this in Chapter 7.) And urging her to eat even less is only going to make her heavier.

The younger she is when she starts dieting, the sooner she may be categorized as obese. In fact, over the last decade, twenty- to twenty-nine-year-old women have experienced one of the greatest increases in obesity.[13] I believe that early dieting is one of the causes of earlier obesity. Of course, a child may already be overweight (because of genetics and/or a sedentary lifestyle) when she starts dieting, but the younger she is when she starts, the more she'll weigh as an adult. One survey showed that when women started dieting in their teen years, their average adult weight was 146 pounds. But when they started in childhood, their average adult weight was 163 pounds[14]—almost twenty pounds more! ***Without dieting, our daughters would be leaner and healthier!***

Even if you've never dieted with your daughter or directly supported her dieting efforts, you still may be encouraging her by your example. As your daughter struggles to identify with you and form her female identity, your dieting practices, eating behaviors, and body image will likely become hers.

DAUGHTER SEE, DAUGHTER DO

My mother dieted every January and June, so I thought that it must be a normal part of womanhood to vow a twenty-pound weight loss with each New Year's resolution and the same twenty-pound loss with each presummer diet.
—*Susie, age 26*

More than half of my focus group participants recalled their mothers controlling their eating in some way—but all of them had vivid memories of their mothers' eating behaviors and body image as they were growing up. They also had a clear awareness of how their mothers' food and body relationship influenced theirs. The greater their mothers' personal investment in dieting and slenderness, the more these adult daughters described their own eating as disordered and their body image as negative.

Called the social learning perspective or passive modeling, a mother's own eating habits and weight concerns serve as modeling cues that a daughter internalizes as her own. Iowa State University found that 81 percent of the fourth graders studied were aware that someone in their family had dieted and 72 percent that someone in their family was worried about being fat.[15] That someone is almost always the mother. And of these same fourth graders, 80 percent had already decided to take on the responsibility of restricting their own eating in some way. Daughter see, daughter do.

The best teachers are those with experience, and we have had a lifetime of experience with dieting. The best students are interested, attentive, and eager for knowledge—and our daughters are absorbing our dieting know-how and becoming experts at the dieting game. The younger you started dieting, the younger your daughter will start dieting. The more diets you've been on, the more diets your daughter will go on. The more severe your weight-loss methods, the more unhealthy hers will be.

YOUR DIETING HISTORY *IS* YOUR DAUGHTER'S DIETING FUTURE.

You can't go back in time and erase your dieting attempts and failures, but you can change your dieting future. You can choose to stop dieting and to set a pro-eating example for your daughter. You can also choose to model healthier eating habits.

YOUR EATING HABITS *ARE* PASSED ALONG TO YOUR DAUGHTER.

If you are a late-night snacker, an emotional eater, or a meal skipper, your daughter is likely to be your eating apprentice. A mother's eating habits set the standard, and a strong relationship exists between a mother's eating habits and her daughter's.

The typical American woman is only eating half of the recommended servings of complex carbohydrates, fruits, and vegetables—and so is the typical daughter. The average mother is consuming 38 percent of her total calories from fat—and so is the average school-age girl.[16] If your diet is high in fat, you most likely provide high-fat foods for your daughter to choose from, and she too has a high-fat diet. What you buy will become your daughter's grocery list and what you eat will become your daughter's food preferences.

Parent/child food likes and dislikes are more strongly correlated with the mother than with the father—and the strongest correlation is between mothers and daughters.[17] What favorite foods do the females in your family share?

My mother and I share a love for many of the same foods. I picture us sitting at her kitchen counter eating thin slices of Genoa salami, rejoicing over handmade Polish kielbasa, or eating a hamburger and french fries at our favorite pub. As you can tell, we both have an affinity for high-fat foods. We also feel a little more permissive sharing our "fat tooth" together—she because her nutritionist daughter is eating it too and me because it's a part of our mother/ daughter food relationship that I enjoy.

Some shared eating habits are memorable and enjoyable to both mothers and daughters, while others can be distressing and negative. Paula's mother was an emotional eater and taught Paula that food was the universal Band-Aid for emotional pain. She always had ten different gallons of ice cream in the freezer, and whenever Paula had a bad day at school or someone hurt her feelings, she would bring her into the kitchen and ask what flavor would make her feel better. Years later, Paula is still trying to decide between chocolate chip and mocha almond fudge and still trying to combat her emotional eating problem.

Daughters mimic not only their mothers' emotional ties to eating and other food behaviors in the kitchen but also their body behaviors in front of the mirror, in the clothes closet, and on the scale. Body dissatisfaction also can be passed down from the mother.

YOUR BODY IMAGE *IS* MIRRORED BY YOUR DAUGHTER.

A correlation exists between a mother's body unhappiness and her daughter's. Mothers who strongly dislike their bodies are more likely to have adolescent daughters who also practice the art of body hatred. And adolescent body discontent persists throughout life. As these young women become adults, they evaluate themselves as larger and less attractive than they actually are. (In comparison, as men grow older, they feel slimmer and more attractive than they really are—and get away with it!)

Here are some of the more subtle yet affecting ways that mothers unknowingly transmit feelings of body dissatisfaction:

- **The Morning Scale Ritual**—"All I know is that the scale is a mean thing. Every time my mother gets on it she becomes very angry and starts using swear words." This mother is teaching her eight-year-old daughter that it is normal for women to get on the scale every morning and get off it feeling angry with themselves and uncomfortable with their bodies.

- **Mirror Avoidance**—"We don't have any full-length mirrors in the house. I asked my mother why and she said it was because she doesn't like looking at her body." Twelve-year-old Mimi shared this with me as well as the fact that she's also gotten used to avoiding the mirror.

- **Bathing Suit Evasion**—"My self-conscious mother never wore a bathing suit at the beach or the pool. She would always come up with some excuse like she forgot it or that she was coming down with a cold." Thirty-year-old Karen is using identical tactics to avoid the bathing suit blues.

- **Body Bashing**—"A day doesn't go by that my mother doesn't call herself fat and ugly." Michelle looks just like her mother, so she has concluded that she must be fat and ugly too.

Some of the saddest tales and statistics are of daughters' memories of their mothers' body image. Of 4,000 daughters surveyed, only 19 percent recall their mothers liking anything about their bodies.[18]

What does this say to a young girl about her own body?

LOVING MOTHERS TEACHING BODY HATRED

My mother once told me that I had long, lovely legs and a short, fat waist. Twenty years later, I still like my legs but curse my waist each and every day.

—Margo, age 35

Once a mother's words are spoken, they are seldom forgotten.

"You're getting a little chunky, aren't you?"

"Pull in your stomach and stand up straight, you'll look thinner."

"Only wear dark colors, they will hide your fat."

"I want you to have a normal life, so please lose some weight."

These comments may be delivered casually by well-meaning moms, but they are far from casual. They are heard as harsh criticisms and stay with us always. In one survey, 55 percent of the daughters said that their mothers were critical of their weights when they were children, 64 percent when they were teens, and 57 percent currently when they are adults.[19] Things don't seem to change much over time.

Some mothers are so critical of their daughters' bodies that they rate their daughters as being even less attractive than their daughters rate themselves.[20] Kathy's mother falls into this category. Kathy calls her mother "her worst weight critic" because she asks about Kathy's weight before asking about her kids, her job, or her health. When her mother greets her, it's not with a hug but with a pinch on the back of the arm to assess her weight. A few years ago, Kathy was going on a tropical vacation with her mother and practically fasted for two weeks before leaving so that she would meet her mother's approval and feel more comfortable in a bathing suit. On their first day at the beach, Kathy came out modeling her new bikini for her mother and exclaiming, "Mom, look at how thin I am!" Instead of praise, her mother responded, "But you still have a stomach, so a one-piece bathing suit would look much better on you." As a result, Kathy has spent many years feeling that something is wrong with her body.

Unfortunately, negative body image is a characteristic shared by millions of women young and old. Only 6 percent of us can say that we honestly like our bodies[21] while the remaining 94 percent avoid mirrors, close-fitting clothing, intimacy, recreation, social functions, and, quite frankly, life because we feel undeserving, uncomfortable, and unsure.

In my seminars for mothers and daughters, one of the questions I ask produces a telling reaction: "What do you like about your body?" I watch the hundreds of women in the room shift uncomfortably in their seats and look down to avoid eye contact. A few women may boldly shout, "I like my breasts!" or "My shapely legs!" but the majority either say nothing or respond more quietly, "I like my eyes" or "My fingernails are okay" or "I guess I like my hair." Their statements, or lack thereof, reflect their deep-rooted discontent with their bodies.

Sometimes I rephrase the question to "What do you dislike about your body?" and it's mayhem. A room full of quiet, modest women becomes a loud, self-deprecating mass shouting in unison what are their most hated body parts. The cry "My thighs!" is usually the most audible. For the fifty-year-old or fifteen-year-old, women's surveys have repeatedly found that the number-one disliked body part is the thighs, followed by the stomach, hips, and buttocks. Incidentally, these are the same parts of the body that make us uniquely feminine and fertile (along with the breasts). Are we really saying that we don't like being women?

I don't think so. I celebrate being a woman every day. Most mothers wish for daughters more than sons and are thrilled when their female lineage is ensured. What we're really saying is that society has caused us to feel uncomfortable with our female bodies.

And mothers, after years of societal influence, are unknowingly teaching their daughters to dislike their natural, womanly body, to fight their internal hunger and fullness signals with external control and dieting, and to become disordered eaters.

MOTHER DOESN'T ALWAYS KNOW BEST

> *It's every mother's responsibility to make sure her daughter has perfect eating habits and a perfect body.*
>
> *—Lonnie, age 45*

Responsibility—it's a consuming word. Mothers have always felt responsible for the way their children "turned out," their value systems, morals, ethics, and health. Now mothers are taking on an additional responsibility—making sure their daughters' bodies "turn out" right.

Based on society's rules and recommendations, you may be doing what you think is best to fulfill this new responsibility of ensuring a thin daughter—but what society tells you to do is at odds with what your daughter's body is telling her to do.

What Society Wants You to Do	What Your Daughter's Body Naturally Wants to Do
Mold her body into an aesthetic ideal	Find a comfortable weight that is biologically and genetically right for her
Encourage dieting	Eat enough food to supply her body with nourishment and fuel
Condition her taste buds	Stimulate all of her taste buds and prefer the taste of sugar starting in infancy, salt starting in the toddler years, and fat starting in adolescence

Feed her low-fat foods	Consume enough fat for brain development and physical growth
Feed her by the clock	Eat when her body tells her it's time to eat
Enforce three balanced meals a day	Snack frequently throughout the day and eat smaller meals
Provide a full-course dinner	Eat a smaller evening snack

Mothers are most surprised to hear that children are usually not hungry at dinnertime and would prefer a small evening snack. Their biological food clocks ring at around four in the afternoon, when their metabolisms are at the peak of calorie burning. Unaware of this metabolic fact, mothers may deny the afternoon snack and instead provide a large, nutritious dinner with all the food groups— and make children sit at the table until they finish all the food on their plate. Of any meal that we or our daughters overeat, dinner is the most likely to be stored. Because the body is preparing for slumber and food needs are minimal, large dinners can cause a quick and steady weight gain. In fact, most women store about one-half of their dinner in their fat cells—because they are overeating. A big dinner meal with large portions is a guaranteed fat cell enlarger. This can happen even if the meal is low fat. By listening to our daughters' food needs and serving them an earlier dinner with perhaps a snack later on, *we would be preventing weight gain!*

Another surprise comes with the knowledge about toddlers' calorie requirements. Everyone's calorie requirement is low at night, but toddlers/preschoolers don't require much food all day long. If you have a daughter between the ages of three and five, her growth rate has slowed down to about four pounds a year, and her appetite, nutrient needs, and calorie requirements have decreased along with it.[22] If she is eating less, it's because she needs less food. Forcing her to eat may create power struggles and may cause her to develop negative attitudes about eating. Without this knowledge, mothers often become frustrated and, as a result, may resort to fear tactics to encourage their daughters to eat more healthfully. Here are a few mothers' comments that five-year-old girls have shared with me:

- "If I don't eat carrots, my mom says I'll go blind."
- "If I don't eat fish, my mother told me that my brain won't work right."
- "My mother said that eating sugar will make my teeth fall out."
- "My mom told me that anyone who eats bacon will get cancer."

Of course these statements are not true, and if you use them, someday your daughter will find out that you were less than honest with her. Be honest with her today, trust her eating instincts, and rise above society's eating rules. This is how we can all become mothers who do know best.

And mothers who know best for their daughters are mothers who know best for themselves. Carol's mother did, and now Carol does. Here is her enlightening story of a healthy generational eating legacy. "My mother didn't care that dieting was in vogue. She never even used the word 'diet,' never controlled my eating habits, and taught me to listen to my body's food messages thirty years ago. I think she intuitively knew that she should let her daughter make her own food decisions. I grew up enjoying food and eating a moderate amount of whatever I wanted. Because of her, I've been at a healthy weight all of my life and have always had a healthy relationship with food. And it's been so easy to have history repeat itself with my daughter. It never even crossed my mind to control her eating. And I'm glad I didn't. She eats little bits of lots of different foods all day long; it's her friends who come over and devour the snack cupboard within minutes." Carol's mother trusted her instincts, taught Carol to do the same, and now Carol is passing this healthy legacy on to her daughter. *Like mother, like daughter can describe a positive food relationship.*

As you are reading through the rest of this book and working toward this more positive mother-daughter food relationship, take the time to acknowledge the immense amount of pressure mothers are under today and the strong devotion they feel toward their daughters.

ACKNOWLEDGING MOTHERS: LITTLE DO DAUGHTERS KNOW

I only wish for a better future for my daughter. I want Jennifer to be thinner so that she will have a life filled with lucrative career opportunities and handsome male prospects.

—*Myra, age 43*

Myra is joined by all mothers whose overriding desire is to provide a better future for their daughters. Many studies have reported that this strong determination is what keeps them going through long days of hard work, stressful jobs, and unmanageable schedules. And it's what keeps them pressuring their daughters to diet and lose weight.

In our society, a "better future" and a slender body are inextricably linked. Both sexes automatically evaluate slender women as being attractive, successful, confident, and happy; whereas overweight women are described as unattractive, unsuccessful, and unhappy. These virtues of thinness and disadvantages of obesity go beyond first impressions to blatant discrimination. The following list documents some of the unfortunate realities of being a fat female in a thin world:

- Overweight females are 40% less likely to go to college.[23]
- Overweight females are 20% less likely to marry.[24]
- Overweight females make $6,700 less a year.[25] (And, of course, regardless of weight, women still make less money than men.)
- Overweight females are more likely to be found guilty by a jury.[26]

Of course we wish for thinner daughters—we want to "save" them from discrimination, poverty, loneliness, and prison. What mother wouldn't?

But in your efforts to "save" your daughter by encouraging dieting, you are only setting her up for a lifetime of weight struggles and health problems. *Dieting is not the solution to life's problems; it can be the cause of obesity, eating disorders, and many health problems.*

With today's documented culture of dieting, you understand why well-intentioned mothers are underfeeding their daughters—but why are some mothers still overfeeding their daughters?

Some deep-rooted reasons may be behind a mother's over-feeding priority. My mother overfed my sister and me because she experienced chronic hunger and witnessed mass starvation in a German work camp during World War II. She wanted to ensure that her daughters never wanted for food. In her heartfelt efforts, she often went overboard with an excess of food in the refrigerator, in the cupboards, and on the table.

Other mothers may not have personally experienced food shortages, but they still want their daughters to be well fed and to grow healthy and strong. Diana's Italian mother would always say "*Mangia, mangia,* you're a growing woman." Diana was fifteen and hadn't grown a millimeter in over two years. She also thought a normal portion size was a half pound of pasta, until she went over to a friend's house for dinner and found out that a half pound was almost enough to serve a family of four. But her mother's motive was well intentioned because she thought that additional food meant additional growth.

Whether it's overfeeding or underfeeding, your choice is based on your personal background and many societal pressures. What's important is that you don't blame yourself or your mother. Instead realize that society is ultimately responsible—*and start doing something differently!*

Disordered eating is a "culture-bound syndrome" unique to Western societies where thinness symbolizes control, liberation, success, beauty, and higher socioeconomic status.[27] If you, your mother, and your daughter lived in a country with different cultural norms and standards of attractiveness, your mother-daughter food relationships would most likely be free of dieting and disordered eating. For example:

- In China, fatness is a symbol of prosperity and longevity.
- In the Arabic culture, female fat is a symbol of fertility and womanhood.
- For the Punjabi Indians, a popular and complimentary greeting is translated to "You look fat and fresh today!"[28]
- The Samoans associate fat with health and wealth, and the typical Samoan mother stands five foot five inches and weighs 200 pounds—and is proud of it![29]

You could pack up your daughter and move to Samoa. But short of that, the reality is that we live in a food- and body-obsessed society whose "lose weight now" message is directed to younger and younger girls at an ever escalating pace.

As a mother in today's society, you have good reason to think you are sincerely trying to protect your daughter by exercising control over her food intake and weight. As a daughter, it's understandable that you initially react with negativism toward your food-controlling mother. But virtually all mothers who are passing the legacy of disordered eating are doing so unknowingly. They, like most women, have been lured into the trap of thinness and dieting with the bait of success, wealth, and health—unaware that they are damaging their own and their daughters' bodies and minds.

To avoid the dieting trap and join the mothers who do know best, read on! The next chapter will make you fully aware of the dangers of dieting and inspire a diet-free mother/daughter food relationship.

CHAPTER THREE

DIETING IS DANGEROUS TO YOUR DAUGHTER'S HEALTH

As *Emily is* getting dressed for school, she notices some changes in her body that she's not happy about: her hips have gotten bigger, her stomach isn't as flat as it used to be, and her jeans are tighter than usual. Determined not to let puberty get the best of her, she vows to do something to keep her body lean and svelte—starting today. Emily walks into the kitchen and informs her mother that she's not eating breakfast because she's starting a one-meal-a-day, fat-busting diet. At first her mother tries to persuade her to have at least some toast, but then she thinks "Why not diet? Maybe if Emily starts dieting now at age twelve, she'll keep her weight down forever and avoid the fifty-pound weight swing I've been dealing with most of my life."

Why not diet? In this chapter I will give you many persuasive reasons why all women should give up dieting and even more powerful reasons why our daughters should never start. Dieting is not a risk-free game of the incredible shrinking woman. It has been linked to such varying health problems as infertility, depression, and hair loss—and has been proven to directly increase the risk for osteo-

porosis and eating disorders. In fact, a young woman who diets is
eight times more likely to develop an eating disorder.[1]

Dieting has become a major public health problem. As the
number of dieting women has escalated over the last three generations, so have the unsettling, potential consequences from dieting.
These include:

fatigue	sleep difficulties
headaches	gallbladder problems
dry skin	thyroid problems
hair loss	hypoglycemia
depression	bone loss
anxiety	reduced maximum height
muscle weakness	constipation
joint pain	mental sluggishness
menstrual irregularities	impaired performance
infertility	weight gain
premenstrual tension	obesity
early menopause	poor body image
electrolyte imbalances	low self-esteem
cold intolerance	eating disorders

You may find this list shocking—because it is! But it reflects
the reality of what we may be doing to ourselves and to our daughters if we encourage them to diet. Luckily, any ill effects attributed
to dieting are 100 percent avoidable—if, of course, we don't diet.
But, as mothers, we're still going full speed ahead with our repeated
dieting attempts, and our daughters have already started their search
for the magical weight-loss formula. Dieting is dangerous to all
women, but our young daughters have the most extensive damage
report because they are dieting during their preadolescent and adolescent years—right when their cells are rapidly dividing, their first
menstrual cycles are starting, and their bodies are maturing into
women.

Half of our daughters are dieting by age nine when the pubertal
transition to womanhood begins, and another third join in over the

next six years when their bodies are in the midst of adolescent development. The adolescent growth spurt is second only to the nine-month prenatal period in its amazing cellular and biological maturation: organs double in size, height and bone strength increase by 20 percent, and female sex hormones introduce themselves for the first time. Along with the growth spurt comes the infamous "fat spurt" where body fat doubles in amount and hips, breasts, buttocks, and thighs begin to take shape.

At least, this is what will happen if your daughter's body is given the proper fuel for the vital growth and fat spurt. When it's deprived nutritionally, a biological battle occurs with many dieting casualties and only one winner. The casualties include bone loss, muscle loss, and hormonal loss. The *only* winner is her fat cells. During adolescence, her fat cells activate to enable her body to mature into a woman's. If she's dieting during this important process, her fat cells will only become stronger, larger, and more active.

I AM WOMAN, HEAR MY FAT CELLS ROAR

I'm trying to help my twelve-year-old daughter lose weight, but she just seems to be getting fatter. Do her fat cells have a mind of their own?

—Fran, age 39

All female fat cells have a mind of their own, but especially those fat cells that come to life during adolescence. They are smart, stubborn, and easily angered when dieting jeopardizes their growth. And they don't just get mad; they get even. In my first book, *Outsmarting the Female Fat Cell*, I explained why you can't starve a female fat cell no matter how hard you try. You may want to review some of the information in that book because it explains how, from puberty through menopause, female fat cells just keep growing, and growing, and growing.

A Fat Cell in Puberty

Through the activation and formation of new fat cells, your daughter's body is programmed with specific instructions to prepare for menstruation, pregnancy, and breast-feeding. Signals are sent to her stomach, hips, thighs—and breasts—to increase the number and size of her fat cells. Her female blueprint calls for a pear-shaped body because extra fat on the lower body is essential for fertility and carrying a developing child for nine months.

It's impossible to disarm this biological programming, although we may try by encouraging our daughters to diet. We assume that helping her to eat less will prevent the formation of new fat cells and shrink their size—but her body is one step ahead of us, anticipating the possibility of a food shortage at this critical stage of development. If your daughter diets, her body responds as if the planet has temporarily run out of fuel and goes into its "red alert" mode to speed up her "get-fat-quick" programming.

For example, instead of producing 5 million fat cells in her left thigh, her body retaliates and increases its inventory to 6 million—just in case. Instead of making her fat cells the size of a dime, her body will make them the size of a quarter. (Don't worry, fat cells are microscopic in size, but the coin comparison helps you to visualize the fat-stimulating effects of dieting.) And instead of developing to be slightly pear-shaped with larger fat cells in the buttocks, hips, and thighs, the increase in the number and size of fat cells will make your daughter extremely pear-shaped with extra-large fat cells.

As I was explaining this to one young daughter, she said, "You mean if I keep dieting, there's a good chance I'll look like an acorn squash instead of a pear, tiny on the top and huge on the bottom?" Not quite, but she may be a larger pear that wears a size-twelve pant or skirt with a size-eight top.

All women have this "get-fat-quick" response when their bodies are threatened with possible starvation, but a young woman is "getting fat quick" during puberty and then "getting fat quicker" when she diets. If we were to view pubertal fat cells under a microscope, this is how they would look with and without dieting:

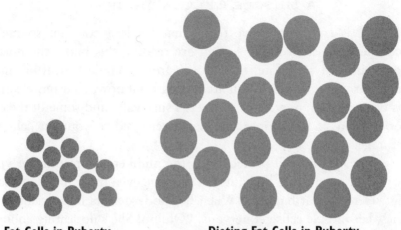

Fat Cells in Puberty   **Dieting Fat Cells in Puberty**

Dieting during adolescence overstimulates the reproduction, growth, and concentration of fat cells in the buttocks, hips, and thighs. It also overstimulates the production of fat storage enzymes so that when your daughter goes off the diet and starts eating again, she'll quickly fill her fat cells to their maximum capacity. In other words, your daughter's body becomes twice as efficient at taking every extra little calorie traveling around in her bloodstream, scooping it up, and storing it in one of her fat cells. Dieting doesn't burn fat, it builds fat and boosts its stubborn, rebellious nature.

"So my daughter's stubborn, rebellious nature extends to her fat cells?" one mother asked. That's one way of thinking about it, but the difference is that unlike volatile mood swings during adolescence, it's not just "a stage" her fat cells are going through, it's a *permanent* change in their disposition.

Perhaps you've had firsthand experience with the long-term effects of dieting on fat cells. Each time you've dieted, you've lost less weight and then gained more back. Unfortunately, much of the weight that you've lost is from muscle tissue, and all of the weight that you've gained back is fat. *Dieting is a fat cell's best friend and a muscle cell's worst enemy.*

47

A MUSCLE CELL IN MOURNING

Muscle is energy-intensive tissue that needs a constant source of calories to sustain itself. As you are reading this book, the muscle on your body is taking the calories from your last meal or snack and burning them up. If you are dieting right now, your muscle mass is being broken down to ensure fat's survival—and some of the calories from your last meal are being rerouted to your fat cells for storage.

Because fat cell protection is the number-one priority of your daughter's maturing body, it will sacrifice even more muscle to save fat. Here's what happens: When her body detects insufficient calories, her muscle cells get nervous. "Oh, no! She's not eating enough. Better hurry and convert some of this muscle to usable fuel so that she can live and breathe."

Think of it this way: *Muscle is expendable; fat is expandable.*

Muscle is metabolically active tissue, so when your daughter's body breaks down muscle mass for needed fuel, her metabolism slows down, and her whole body (except for her fat cells) goes into the energy-saving mode. She's taking in less energy, so her body conserves it to adjust to the food shortage. For example, if she's eating only 1,000 calories, her metabolism will try to compensate by decreasing her caloric needs to 1,000 calories. And the longer she diets and the greater her weight loss, the slower her metabolism will be. Once her metabolism has been lowered, it may never return to normal—unless she stops dieting.

A lower-than-normal metabolism means that all of your daughter's cells and organs will work sluggishly. As her digestive system slows down, she may start complaining of constipation. As her thyroid gland slows down, she may start noticing more fatigue and lethargy. As her brain slows down, she may notice an inability to concentrate, and you may notice a drop in her grades. Studies have shown that dieters do not perform as well in school. They think more slowly, react more slowly, and may experience short-term memory loss. So, if she "forgets" to take out the trash, it may be that her starving brain is too busy sending signals for fat storage—and sending signals to hurry up and start eating high-calorie foods again. Her brain has had enough of the carrot sticks and skinless chicken breast and urges her to bring on the chocolate, cheesecake, and chips.

A Brain Cell in Starvation

During puberty, the appetite center and reproductive center in a woman's brain form a lifelong partnership. While the reproductive center is transmitting the order to multiply and enlarge the fat cells for the life-giving functions of pregnancy and breast-feeding, the appetite center is sending powerful signals to increase the desire for high-calorie fat and sugar foods for the assurance of fat cell growth. Like female fat cells, the female preference for fat and sugar is activated at puberty and permanently ingrained in our biological makeup.

Dieting during puberty will only make your daughter's fat-stimulating reproductive center and fat-loving appetite center work overtime. Instead of subtly requesting some chocolate or ice cream, her appetite center will demand a pound of chocolate or a gallon of ice cream to make up for the scarcity of food.

Historically, whenever food has been scarce, people have become preoccupied with food as a survival mechanism. During famines, drought, and food shortages, our brains are designed to think about and desire food, our bodies to search for food, and our taste buds to salivate more when we do find food. The same holds true with a self-imposed food shortage—except the brain, taste buds, and body are in a state of confusion. The brain sees food, knows it's plentiful, but you're not eating. Puzzled by your failure to devour the needed calories in those freshly baked cookies within arm's reach, your brain first checks your vision to make sure everything is still working properly, then it demands that you eat the cookies by increasing your appetite and decreasing your willpower.

Lack of willpower is the most common obstacle to dieting cited by women.[2] How can any woman have willpower when her body is going through these reactions? *Dieting triggers a biological response to overeat.*

Depriving your body of food is like depriving your body of oxygen—an unnatural state that causes overcompensation. When you hold your breath until your body forces you to breathe, your rate of breathing increases for a while to compensate for the oxygen deprivation. The same is true of dieting; your body will force you to increase your calorie intake to compensate for the food deprivation.

The next time you are presented with a new, guaranteed weight-loss diet, resist the temptation because you now know the only guaranteed results will be larger, more stubborn fat cells, less muscle, a higher intake of fat and sugar, and weight gain. If your daughter wakes up tomorrow morning and informs you that she's starting a new diet, inform her that her body's built-in save-the-fat, antistarvation defense mechanisms will immediately start to fight against her efforts—and win by making her lose at the dieting game.

Save-the-Fat Defense System

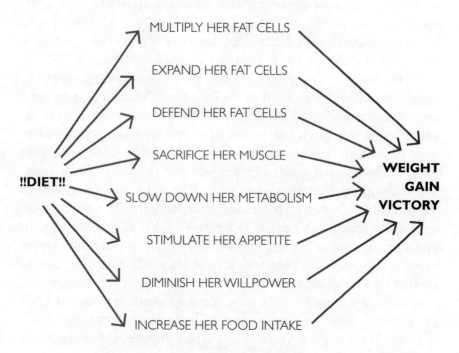

Even if she does lose some weight with dieting, it's a temporary loss. As soon as she goes off the diet, her slower metabolism, increased fat-storing efficiency, and increased desire for high-calorie foods all ensure that she will regain the weight—plus some, and sometimes plus a lot.

Today I counseled a young woman who weighed 130 pounds when she started dieting six years ago; now, after six major diets and many minidiets (as she called them), she weighs 215 pounds. She started at Nutrisystem at age thirteen, then went to Diet Center, then Jenny Craig, then Weight Watchers—then at age eighteen went to Optifast. Now she is battling bulimia. As she put it, "I couldn't take it any longer. Every time I dieted, I would feel lousy, hate myself, binge, and then hate myself more. I was so frustrated that I didn't know what else to do, so I started throwing up." Her case is not uncommon; three out of every four bulimics report that the inability to stay on a diet led to bingeing and then eventually to purging.[3]

THE DIETING BACKLASH: FROM DISORDERED EATING TO EATING DISORDERS

My mother put me on my first diet at age eight, I was anorexic in high school, bulimic in college, and obese for my twenty-fifth birthday.

—Jan, age 32

Mothers, listen to this: A dieting daughter is *eight times* more likely to suffer from an eating disorder than a daughter who has never dieted.[4]

Over a dozen recent studies point to dieting as the most common and most predictable cause of eating disorders. At the highly acclaimed eating disorder clinic, The Renfrew Center in Philadelphia, 88 percent of eating disorder patients, both anorexic and bulimic, cited prolonged dieting as the number-one factor leading to their illness.[5] **Dieting is a major risk factor for eating disorders!!**

What begins as an innocent attempt to lose weight can result in a serious eating disorder. It did with me. Like most women of my generation, I started dieting in high school. I skipped meals and cut calories to get down to my initial weight goal of 120 pounds, but when I got there, the hoped-for pot of gold was not awaiting me at the end of the dieting rainbow. Therefore, I concluded that 120 must not be the magical number and kept dieting, and dieting, and dieting—until I reached 99 pounds. I might have kept dieting and losing weight had I not left for college and started eating again as a way to cope with the stress of this life transition.

Dieting started me down the path of developing an eating disorder, and it appears that today far too many young women are also journeying down this well-traveled road. The University of Minnesota's Adolescent Health Program studied the dieting behaviors of 36,000 students in grades seven through twelve and found that the chronic dieters (those who were dieting at least ten times a year) were[6]:

10 times more likely to vomit 1 or more times a week.

8 times more likely to use ipecac to induce vomiting.

7 times more likely to use laxatives to induce diarrhea.

7 times more likely to use diuretics to dehydrate the body.

Just think how much healthier these young women would be if they didn't feel compelled to be thin. They wouldn't be vomiting or abusing laxatives and diuretics—and they wouldn't be on the road to developing an eating disorder.

Dieting causes a domino effect. It leads to bingeing, subsequent dieting attempts, drastic weight-loss techniques, disordered eating, and then eating disorders. I have witnessed this predictable progression of events with many young women. Sometimes it can take years; other times it's only a matter of days. With Martha, her first diet led to her first binge, which led immediately to her first purge with laxatives. She started with a standard high-protein diet on her twelfth birthday, and four days later she found herself bingeing on leftover birthday cake. Consumed with the fear of gaining weight, she took three of her mother's laxatives and within three months was taking over twenty laxatives a day. Eventually, her colon was beyond repair, and after part of it was surgically removed, she started to gain weight quickly. She fasted, then started bingeing again, and finally resorted to vomiting—first once a day and then five times a day. For Martha, one seemingly safe diet led to twenty laxatives a day and five visits a day to the "porcelain god" (as she and other bulimics call the toilet). It may take only five diets or as many as fifty, but these are the potential consequences of your daughter's continual dieting.

If your daughter is anorexic or bulimic, I urge you to find an experienced, licensed therapist who uses a multidisciplinary team approach with a nutritionist, physician, psychiatrist, and exercise physiologist. Far too often, failure to recover from an eating disorder is due to an inadequate treatment process. Some eating disorder specialists still use weigh-ins and calorie counting in treatment, but these only "feed" into the patient's already obsessive behaviors. Ask around for referrals, get recommendations from the national eating disorder organizations, and get your daughter expert help. (You can also refer to Chapter 7 for further guidance.)

If your daughter is actively dieting, don't wait until she becomes an eating disorder victim. She may be closer than you think. There is a fine line between the estimated 80 percent of our daughters who are disordered eaters and the 10 percent who have eating disorders.[7] Take a look at the comparison of the diagnostic criteria for anorexia and the common characteristics of today's dieting daughters:

Diagnostic Criteria for Anorexia[8]	Characteristics of Dieting Daughters
Intense fear of becoming overweight	80% fear weight gain[9]
Disturbance in body image	82% of those at a normal weight think they are too fat[10]
Refusal to maintain weight at 85% of a healthy normal weight	Average desired weight is at 86.5% of healthy normal weight for height[11]

This comparison is a little too close for comfort. As you can see, anorexia is now more a matter of degree than a matter of diagnosis. Many of our daughters are "near anorexics"; they exhibit some of the characteristic behaviors and attitudes, but not quite enough of them for a clinical diagnosis . . . yet. However, they are caught somewhere in the disordered eating continuum and moving down the path toward one or the other of its devastating ends.

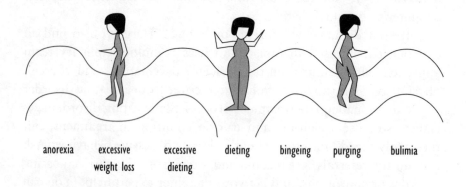

anorexia   excessive   excessive   dieting   bingeing   purging   bulimia
            weight loss   dieting

Dieting is the number-one factor that sets this continuum in motion. Without dieting, fewer women would be on the path to eating disorders.

Bulimia is at the other end of the continuum from anorexia, and like anorexia, its manifestations vary in degree. The classic description of bulimia is bingeing on excessive amounts of food (up to 30,000 calories have been documented!) and purging through vomiting at least two times a week. (Some women vomit more than three times a day.) But a binge is relative—it can be as large as five packages of cookies or as small as an extra stalk of broccoli. Bingeing is overeating in *any* amount—and overeating leads to fear of weight gain that can then lead to purging. Purging now takes many forms besides vomiting. In fact, research has shown that dieting is the most common method of purging today.[12] Think about it: Dieting is the primary cause of bulimia, *and* dieting is the most common purging method that reinforces the bulimic behavior and propels the destructive binge/purge cycle.

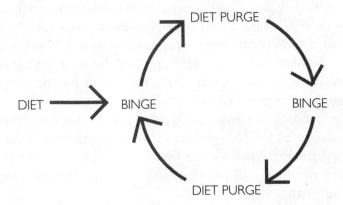

Without realizing it, many of us and our daughters may "purge" through dieting or other means after we've overeaten. How would you complete this sentence: I ate too much at dinner, so I need to:

a. skip breakfast tomorrow

b. go on a restrictive diet tomorrow

c. fast for the next twenty-four hours

d. exercise for three hours to "burn off" the extra calories

e. take some laxatives

f. go into the bathroom to vomit

g. eat a whole package of cookies because I've blown it

If none of the options described your reaction to the overeating scenario and instead your response was "Oh, well, I overate. One meal of overindulgence is not going to cause any permanent weight gain," congratulations! And if you don't have a daughter, find someone else's and take her under your healthy wing.

Certainly, some of these listed choices are more harmful than others, but all are purging behaviors (except g, which is a form of bingeing). All are also signs of disordered eating on the verge of becoming an eating disorder. Even exercise, the most positive, health-promoting behavior we can incorporate into our lives, can be a major health problem when it is taken to the extreme. After some women eat, they figure out exactly how much and how long they need to exercise to burn up the calories before they take hold. I've counseled a ten-year-old who was exercising two hours a day, a fourteen-year-old who was exercising four hours a day, and a fifteen-year-old who was running marathons—all for the purpose of exercising away unwanted calories.

This amount of exercise is excessive and unhealthy. Some call it an exercise addiction; others call it hypergymnasia; I call it an *exercise disorder.* When we are overexercising for the sole purpose of ridding our bodies of calories, it is a disorder that must be identified and treated.

How can you tell if your daughter (or you) has an exercise disorder? There are three warning signs:

1. She must work out five to seven days a week for at least two hours per session, even if she is ill or injured.

2. She organizes her life around exercise at the expense of friendships, family activities, and school activities.

3. She feels guilty when she misses a workout and can't seem to let go of the guilt.

Far too often, overexercise and undereating go hand-in-hand. This combination is so stressful to a woman's body that it may have no other option than to stop or diminish such essential female functions as estrogen production and monthly blood flow. When a woman stops menstruating, her estrogen levels plummet and all of her cells are deprived of estrogen. Her skin becomes dry, and her hair and her bones become brittle. Even with normal menstrual cycles, overexercised, dieting women may have lower than normal estrogen levels and weaker than normal bone strength. Because bone loss may be irreversible, it is one of the more devastating effects of dieting.

A BONE TO PICK WITH DIETING

I knew I was finally in shape and thin enough when my periods stopped.

—Linda, age 19

I knew Linda's bones were in bad shape *because* her periods had stopped and her estrogen level was quickly declining. The female sex hormone, estrogen, is the gatekeeper for a woman's bone mass. Estrogen helps us to absorb calcium and deposit calcium in our bones. Both dieting and overexercise can reduce blood estrogen levels and cause either a complete cessation of the menstrual cycle or some type of menstrual irregularity. Any way you look at it, dieting is not good for a woman's bone mass or menstrual cycle. Period.

Because dieting during adolescence can result in permanently weak, porous bones characteristic of osteoporosis, it requires a special, bold-faced warning. The USDA Children's Research Center recently released news that made headlines across the country. Peak bone formation begins at puberty with the surge of estrogen and ends at about age fifteen; in females, almost no new bone is formed after the age of twenty-five.[13] Because the amount of bone deposited during puberty determines your daughter's risk for osteoporosis for the rest of her life, she may be literally dieting away her bones and missing out on a once-in-a-lifetime opportunity to build bone density and reduce the risk of fractures caused by osteoporosis.

Young girls today are starting their first diets at age eight or nine, right when the intensive effort for bone laying begins, and as many as 80 percent are dieting between the bone formative years of eight and fifteen.[14] This means that four out of five young women may be jeopardizing their bone health. The stress of dieting by itself will rob strength from bone tissue, but inadequate calcium intake also comes with dieting. And as you know, calcium plays an important role in bone health.

Few, if any, dieting women would choose a glass of milk over a diet soft drink. Their rationale makes sense from a calorie standpoint. Why consume almost 200 calories when you can have zero, none, *nada*—and the taste of sugar? But from a bone health standpoint, the choice makes no sense at all. Milk products are one of the major sources of calcium, while the phosphorous found in soft drinks (both diet and regular, but there's more in diet) may reduce calcium absorption. Not only will your daughter be deficient in calcium, but she will also be absorbing less of what she does consume. How many diet soft drinks does your daughter drink a day? Young women under the age of eighteen constitute one of the fastest-growing groups of diet soft drink consumers and one of the fastest-dwindling groups of milk consumers. Not a good ratio.

According to national nutrition surveys, 50 to 84 percent of adolescent girls are not getting the 1,200 mg of calcium they need daily. Because the majority of adult bone mass is laid down during the adolescent years, research has shown that adult women who had calcium-poor diets in their teen years had a significantly lower bone mass than their calcium-rich counterparts—and a significantly higher risk of bone fractures (up to 50 percent higher) later in life.[15]

If your daughter is dieting, inadequate calcium, calories, and estrogen will ensure not only that her bones will be weaker than normal but that she will also be shorter than normal. Growing daughters need to increase their bone strength to prevent fractures *and* increase their bone length to reach their maximum height. Dieting can stunt your daughter's height by cutting her adolescent growth rate in half.[16] If the threat of porous, weak bones doesn't motivate your daughter to stop dieting, the possibility of reduced maximum height may be highly motivating. All young women I spoke with wanted to do everything they possibly could to grow as tall as they possibly could—and this information persuaded them to stop dieting.

Human bone can withstand quite a lot—24,000 pounds of stress per square inch (for comparison, steel can only withstand 6,000 pounds of stress), but the stress of dieting and overexercising is just too much for the bone to handle.

Premature osteoporosis will strike one out of every two women. Dieting is partly responsible for this current women's health problem because once bone tissue is lost, it may never come back as dense and strong. Even with calcium supplements and estrogen replacement, women are still breaking hips and collapsing their spinal columns. As our daughters are starting to diet at younger ages, the future incidence of osteoporosis is predicted to rise even higher. Already some twenty-year-old women have premature osteoporosis, and as they mature and reach menopause, they will have less bone to lose and, therefore, will suffer more devastating effects from osteoporosis. *Prevention is the only solution to osteoporosis. It must begin before adolescence and must include a diet-free lifestyle.*

After hearing about the strong link between dieting and bone loss, mothers are extremely concerned and want to do something to help their daughters. The first question I ask them is: "Are you doing *anything* to encourage your daughter to diet?"

One mother emphatically answered, "No!! I don't diet, and I don't pressure my daughter to diet. She diets on her own." Then I asked her, "Are you doing anything to help your daughter lose weight?" and she talked nonstop for fifteen minutes about the low-fat diet she's put her whole family on, her low-fat recipes, nonfat snacks, and no-fat rules.

I think it's time to define "a diet."

A DIET IS A DIET IS A DIET

My daughter and I gave up dieting a couple of years ago. We're strict vegetarians now and eat only ten grams of fat a day.

—Teresa, age 39

This *is* dieting; it's just disguised as being a lifestyle change. Teresa and her daughter had become very-low-fat vegetarians as a speedy solution to weight loss—and they are not alone. About one-fifth of us and one-third of our daughters report following a vegetarian diet.[17] Some choose it for philosophical or health reasons, but others choose to eliminate animal foods as a way to cut calories. One aspiring comedienne put a different twist on vegetarian diets when she told me, "I've become a vegetarian not because I love animals but because I hate plants." For her, though, becoming a vegetarian was a way to limit her food intake without having to say she was dieting.

As awareness has increased on the failure rate of dieting, we "say" that we have given it up for a healthy lifestyle. But have we really? We may no longer be on traditional low-calorie diets, but instead we're on low-fat "diets," low-sugar "diets," exercise "diets," or vegetarian "diets." We still have the diet mentality—following a structured plan, counting the grams of fat, depriving ourselves of favorite foods, and getting on the scale to see how much weight we've lost. Then, if the numbers on the scale don't meet our approval, we cut even more fat and sugar just as we would cut calories.

One set of weight-loss rules has just replaced another. We're not supposed to cut calories, so we're cutting fat. We're not supposed to be eating less, so we're exercising more. All to produce a calorie deficit and quick weight loss. I call this *pseudodieting*—and many women are doing it and encouraging this new type of dieting in their daughters.

While researching *Like Mother, Like Daughter*, I stood on a street corner in downtown Oakland, California, during the lunch hour. With clipboard in hand, I randomly stopped women and asked them if they were currently doing anything to lose weight. Although 30 percent acknowledged that they were following a traditional low-calorie diet, a whopping 99 percent said that they were doing one or more of the following:

- *Cutting out* much of the fat from their diets
- *Buying only* nonfat foods
- *Eating only* fruits, vegetables, and whole grains
- *Eliminating* high-fat snacks and desserts
- *Staying away* from processed sugar
- *Giving up* their favorite high-fat foods

Most of their responses centered around reducing the fat content of their diets, but their restrictive choice of words reveals that they were striving to cut their fat intake unrealistically low—and, therefore, dieting.

According to the Food Marketing Institute, 60 percent of those surveyed say that fat is now their primary nutrition concern when making food choices.[18] A decade ago, only 8 percent were evaluating foods based on the fat content. I'm thrilled that we are more conscious about fat, but I'm also concerned that we and our daughters are going overboard. With thousands of reduced-fat and fat-free foods introduced over the last few years, we are becoming lipohysteric (*lipo* means fat) mothers and our daughters are becoming fatphobic females, mainly to lose weight. One thirteen-year-old shared with me that she doesn't eat bread any longer because she discovered it contained one gram of fat per serving.

Our daughters are more extreme in their fat reductions and more knowledgeable about the fat content of foods than we are. They are excellent sleuths at identifying foods high in fat (or even foods that contain any fat) and precise scientists in evaluating the fat content of their diets. For some, their nutritional awareness may surpass their awareness of current events. At Arizona State University, a pop quiz revealed some unnerving answers from students who thought Alzheimer's was an imported beer, Sandra Day O'Connor an actress on *L.A. Law,* and OSHA a killer whale at Sea World.[19] Our daughters may be spending more time reading the fat grams on food labels than reading newspapers or textbooks.

Let me shed some "lite" on the topic of very-low-fat diets.

If we or our daughters do not consume enough fat, we may become deficient in fat-soluble vitamins, essential fatty acids, natural body oils, and vital female hormones. (Estrogen is made from fat.) We may also trigger the starvation response to increase fat storage through a reduction in metabolism and an increase in appetite— and, thus, experience the enigma of *low-fat weight gain.*

A frustrated young woman entered my office, sat herself down on the couch, and before introducing herself said, "Something is wrong with me. I've been eating nonfat foods for the last six months and have gained four pounds. What's happening?" Her food records uncovered that she was eating only eight grams of fat a day—but overeating such nonfat foods as nonfat frozen yogurt, bagels, fruit, and rice cakes. She wasn't eating enough fat, which threatened her fat cells, and she was eating too much starch, fruit, and other nonfat foods, which made her fat cells pleasantly plump.

It simply isn't true that you can eat anything you want, in any quantity you want, whenever you want, as long as it's nonfat. Overeating nonfat foods will lead to weight gain.

And it appears that many are overeating nonfat foods. When we eat nonfat or low-fat, we often compensate by overeating. This has always been my theory, and researchers at Pennsylvania State University have recently proven it. Groups of women were given either low-fat or regular yogurt for breakfast. Those women who didn't know which type of yogurt they were eating ate moderately throughout the day. But those who were told that they were eating low-fat yogurt (even if it was the regular version) ate more of everything else all day long.[20] Their perception of the fat content directed their eating habits and justified overeating.

Eating very low fat can be a form of dieting that will stimulate our desire for more food, reduce our metabolisms, and activate the fat cells on our buttocks, hips, and thighs. Don't be fooled; many diets are now being camouflaged as healthy eating plans and behavior change programs. Like many of the weight-loss programs, Weight Watchers has redesigned its program to a lifestyle approach, but the weigh-ins are still there and the postdiet weight gain still occurs. Some women have argued with me that Weight Watchers isn't really a diet because they've been on it six times, and it's worked for them every single time. My question to them is: "Then why did you have to join six times?"

If the primary motivation for any weight-loss plan is quick loss, then it's a diet and bound to fail. My intent is not to pick on Weight Watchers. To the contrary, out of all the franchised weight-loss programs, I feel that Weight Watchers is the healthiest and safest—as long as the goal is slow, permanent weight loss.

It doesn't matter what name or form a diet takes; what does matter is that you are depriving yourself and/or your daughter and are trying to "lose weight" or "burn fat" quickly. Whether it's a fad diet, diet pill, camouflaged diet, or pseudodiet, *if you can't see yourself eating this way for the rest of your life, then it's a diet.*

Can you see yourself eating no fat for the rest of your life?

Can you imagine yourself exercising every day for the rest of your life?

Can you live without your favorite foods for the rest of your life?

If the answer to these questions is "no," then you're dieting, triggering the starvation response, setting the disordered eating dominos in motion, and jeopardizing your physical—and psychological—health.

The bad news about dieting isn't over yet.

DIETS SHOULD CARRY WARNING LABELS

I wish that I had never started dieting. I thought I was fat when I first started dieting, but now I would give anything to have my prediet body back. Over the last ten years, I've put on fifty pounds, become preoccupied with weight, self-conscious, and insecure. Why didn't anyone warn me about dieting before I started?

—*Norma, age 25*

Most women I come in contact with have the same wish. They may still wish for a thinner body, but they wish they had never chosen dieting as their method. They realize that dieting is one of the major contributors of their self-consciousness, poor body image, and low self-esteem. No one could have warned Norma or you about the negative psychological effects of dieting because no one knew about them. But now we know—and you *can* warn your daughter.

Dieting leads to weight and food preoccupation, obsessions with the scale, feelings of failure, fears of weight gain, and poor body image. Dieting and its resulting body dissatisfaction are not reserved for the overweight. Studies have shown that just as many underweight and normal-weight women as those who are overweight are dieting their way to body dissatisfaction. Of the twelve-to twenty-three-year-old women studied, 82 percent who desired to lose weight were *not* overweight[21]—but they were dieting and unhappy with their bodies just the same.

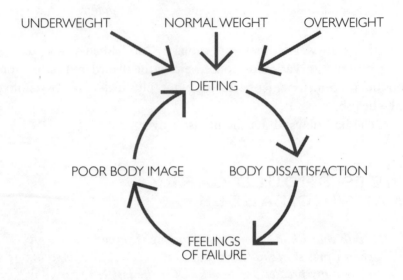

The culture of dieting has caused women of every weight category to become caught in a downward spiral of body dissatisfaction and poor body image. And unfortunately, women of every age category have become caught in it as well. The landmark 1991 American Association of University Women (AAUW) study, "Short-changing Girls, Shortchanging America," was shocking in its findings about poor body image and low self-esteem: at the young age of nine, only 60 percent of the 3,000 girls surveyed said that "they were happy with who they are," and by the time these girls completed puberty and reached their teen years, a mere 29 percent expressed contentment with who they were.[22] In another equally disturbing study, the majority of ten-year-olds surveyed rated themselves as "the single least attractive" girl in their class.[23] Young girls and young women are battling body image and self-esteem issues most of us never dreamed of at their ages.

What is happening to our young daughters? Mary Pipher, in her best-selling book, *Reviving Ophelia*, describes this mass unhappiness as a "hurricane" to alert us to the deep problems of young girls today that stem in part from their vulnerability to cultural pressures and norms that focus on appearance.[24]

Appearance now defines happiness for *both* women and girls. And what is the number-one determining aspect of appearance? Weight. What is the primary method to lose weight? Dieting. What is the outcome of dieting? Body dissatisfaction, disordered eating, eating disorders, and obesity.

Most of us became aware of cultural standards of attractiveness in our teen years, but our daughters have absorbed this kind of definition of beauty by age six.[25] They describe thinner women as beautiful and prefer to associate themselves with thinner friends. As they mature, they start to compare their bodies to countless slender media images that they have come to idolize and value. I spoke with a maturing nine-year-old who summarized her strife in one sentence: "Every beautiful girl in cartoons, TV shows, or the movies is thin, but I'm getting fat, which means I'm getting ugly." What were you thinking about at age nine? How you could be thinner, or how you could fit in one more game before your mother called you in for the night?

Young girls are not taught how the female body must develop to be psychologically and physiologically healthy; rather they are taught how the female body must look to be perceived as beautiful. Thus, by the teen years, 71 percent are not happy with who they are, 82 percent are not happy with how they look, 80 percent are dieting, and 10 percent have an eating disorder. Our daughters' future will be marked with compromised physical and psychological health—*unless we educate them and actively serve as healthier role models!*

In one mother's effort to spread the word about the dangers of dieting, she printed some warning signs on her computer and passed them out to her daughters, her daughters' friends, neighborhood mothers, the PTA, and other organizations. This was her sign:

> ### WARNING:
>
> Dieting during puberty, the childbearing years, and any other time in a woman's life may cause severe physical damage and psychological harm.

You can undo the damage from dieting. It's not too late for yourself—and it's definitely not too late for you to make some important pro-eating, anti-dieting changes in your mother/daughter food relationship.

If your daughter proclaims, "I'm starting a diet today," whether it's a traditional diet or a camouflaged diet, what she is really saying is "I'm going on a diet-induced path to disordered eating that will likely lead to low self-esteem, health problems, obesity, and/or an eating disorder."

Do everything within your power to convince her otherwise. But be prepared to vie against other powerful players advocating thinness and pressuring her to diet. Unless you never allow your daughter to watch television, buy a magazine, or go out of the house again, you can't control her exposure to these influences—but you can educate her, share with her your personal experiences, and make her aware of the unhealthy trap of dieting.

One of the most effective ways to avoid the trap of dieting is through a full understanding of the biological realities of the female body and an appreciation of the many ways fat can benefit a woman from puberty through menopause. Female fat is not an enemy but an ally—ensuring fertility, the wonderful functions of pregnancy and breast-feeding, a lower risk of heart disease, and a longer, healthier life.

CHAPTER FOUR

FROM GIRLHOOD TO WOMANHOOD: THE HEALTHY BIOLOGICAL PASSAGE

As *Stephanie blows* out the thirteen candles on her birthday cake, her smile fades to a look of confusion. She's not sure if she wants to become a "teenager" because everything is changing: her friendships, her moods, her weight, her body. "What is there to celebrate?" she ponders. "Periods, pounds, and PMS? I can't eat this birthday cake anyway because it will only make me fatter than I already am." Two other women are looking at the cake before them with the same anxious feelings about their bodies. Her mother has just had another child and is struggling to lose the weight she gained during pregnancy, and her grandmother is menopausal and has recently declared war against her expanding waistline. Each of them decides to pass on the cake.

These three generations of women may be in different stages of the female lifecycle—puberty, postpregnancy, and menopause—but they all share the same body concerns and weight frustrations and are asking the same perplexing questions: Why is my body changing even though my eating habits and activity level haven't? Why isn't my body cooperating with my weight-loss efforts? Why is my body betraying me?

Instead of embracing these passages through womanhood, many are conflicted about them. This internal discord is caused partly by the false expectations society sets up for the maturing woman. The image of this woman looks almost prepubescent, is unrealistically thin, manages to emerge from childbirth without left-over pounds, loose skin, or stretch marks, then travels through menopause with no visible changes in body shape, tone, or weight. Where are these women? I don't personally know of any, but, nevertheless, we believe that this ageless, changeless, always-thin woman not only exists but is someone we can and should pattern ourselves after. If it appears, however, that a model, celebrity, or next-door neighbor is passing through life's transitions untouched, rest assured that she has probably been touched plenty—by plastic surgeons, liposuction needles, cosmetologists, and personal trainers. She may also be one of the fortunate few to be endowed with favorable genes (at least favorable by society's standards).

This unrealistic portrayal of womanhood also reflects a lack of understanding, appreciation, and acceptance of the stages of female passage. Because we are not fully aware of the physiological changes that must occur during puberty, pregnancy, and menopause, we feel betrayed by our bodies and thus become trapped in weight preoccupation, poor body image, and low self-esteem. As the intellectual pioneer Simone DeBeauvoir perceptively observed, "to lose confidence in one's body is to lose confidence in one's self."[1]

To restore confidence in ourselves and to regain respect for our bodies, we and our daughters must reclaim an appreciation for our biological rites of passage through puberty, pregnancy, and menopause—or, as I call them, *biological rights of passage.* Our daughters are entitled to certain rights during puberty, and we are entitled to certain rights during pregnancy and menopause. And by reclaiming these rights, we can feel empowered instead of betrayed; we can feel at peace with the natural physiological changes that accompany these special times in our lives.

The need to understand and appreciate the wonders of the female body is most urgent with our young daughters. Many are entering puberty at odds with their hormones and engaged in a futile battle with their fat cells. Young girls and boys share this prevailing negative attitude toward the female body; both view female pubescent changes as negative, but male changes as positive. Adolescent boys have an increase in muscle mass and wet dreams (perhaps embarrassing but, nonetheless, pleasurable); adolescent girls have an increase in body fat and begin menstruation, neither of which is viewed as pleasurable. Unfortunately, these negative attitudes are guiding our young daughters through adolescence.

WHAT LITTLE GIRLS ARE REALLY MADE OF

I don't want to start my period. I'll just get pimples on my face, fat on my thighs, and blood on my underwear.
—Kitty, age 9

Adolescence has always been a time of turmoil. We may have felt unprepared for the physical and emotional changes in our bodies and minds during puberty, but our daughters are even less prepared because they are entering puberty at younger ages. In 1877, the average age of menarche (the first menstrual cycle) was 14.75; by 1947, the average age had dropped to 12.8.[2] Today, the majority of young women have started their periods by age 12. And the first developmental changes of puberty actually begin two to four years *before* the first menstrual cycle. This means that many eight- and nine-year-old girls are dealing with the beginnings of womanhood: female hormones, an increase in body fat, and the formation of hips and breasts. How mentally or emotionally prepared can a third, fourth, or fifth grader be for these dramatic changes?

Theories abound for why puberty and menarche are occurring at increasingly younger ages. Some believe the reason lies in better nourishment; others that an increase in height is an influential factor; some that global electricity has stimulated an early release of hormones; and still others that the hormones added to chicken and beef have activated the reproductive system prematurely. It may be a combination of these factors, but regardless of the causes, the trend toward earlier menarche continues—emphasizing the need for a strong, supportive mother-daughter relationship and the importance of an early preparation of our daughters for puberty.

If our daughters are not adequately prepared to accept the body changes during puberty, they may be more vulnerable to disordered eating. A study of middle-school females confirms a predictable sequence of events that begins with a negative response to the body changes during puberty and ends with disordered eating.[3]

BODY CHANGES $\rightarrow$ BODY DISSATISFACTION $\rightarrow$ DESIRE THINNESS $\rightarrow$ DIETING $\rightarrow$ DISORDERED EATING

How can we, as concerned mothers, alter this unhealthy response to puberty? We can't stop the body changes, but through education, awareness, and realistic expectations, we can prepare our daughters and modify their attitudes surrounding these changes. By doing so, the sequence of events will instead be:

BODY CHANGES $\rightarrow$ BODY ACCEPTANCE

and we will make a major step toward abolishing body hatred, the pursuit of thinness, dieting, disordered eating, and eating disorders.

Your role is vital. You can help your daughter anticipate the changes and feel comfortable with her female development during puberty and beyond. Because puberty begins at a younger age, and body image is set in puberty and remains relatively constant throughout life, the earlier you start to prepare your daughter for her changes, the better. *Psychology Today* surveyed 33,000 adult women and found that those who currently had positive body images remembered themselves as also having positive body images in their adolescent years.[4]

Think back to your own experience with adolescence and puberty. Were you prepared for the changes in your body? What did your mother do (or not do) to prepare you? What do you wish she

70

had done differently? One interviewee answered, "I was so unprepared that I thought some disease was making me fat and irritable. I had no idea what was going on in my body, and it wasn't until I became pregnant that I finally came to terms with the fat-storing power of estrogen. My mother didn't even talk about menstruation, she just gave me a box of pads and told me to talk to my older sister. I wish she had taken my hand and guided me with her experience and wisdom." Whatever you feel was missing from your developmental years, do your best to provide it for your daughter—and inform her of her *biological rights of passage.*

AN ADOLESCENT'S BIOLOGICAL RIGHT OF PASSAGE

Wait a minute, Mom. Are you telling me that this one little hormone estrogen does all that stuff in a woman's body? That's really neat!

—Jessica, age 12

What follows is a discussion that you won't typically find in biology textbooks or women's magazines. Many books describe the stages of puberty and some of the physiological changes, but they don't explain the changes as they pertain to fat cell physiology, body respect, and body appreciation. I have written this section in such a way that your daughter can easily understand her biological rights of passage: her right to be at peace with estrogen, fat cells, and the menstrual cycle. You may want to give this book to her, use my words, or try to explain her rights in a way that may be more comfortable for you.

BIOLOGICAL RIGHT #1—BE EMPOWERED BY ESTROGEN

Estrogen is a life-enhancing, life-extending hormone. When the first molecules of estrogen are released, a young girl's body and mind undergo a miraculous transformation. Every single cell in her body has been awaiting this unique hormone, and each is thankful for estrogen's life-giving properties.

- Bone cells start to use the estrogen to increase strength and resiliency.

- Special liver cells are activated and start manufacturing the "good" cholesterol that scrubs arteries clean and lowers the risk of heart attacks for many years. Even at age sixty, men are almost four times more likely than women to have a heart attack because they have not been granted the protective effects of estrogen.[5]

- Breast cells come to life and provide the ability to breast-feed children.

- Uterine and ovarian cells mature and start releasing the eggs for fertilization and preparing the home for the developing baby.

- Skin cells are stimulated to secrete natural oils that keep the skin healthy.

- Brain cells are prompted to release mood-enhancing chemicals that keep her sensitive to her surroundings and receptive to her emotional needs.

and . . .

- Fat cells are activated and directed to expand, multiply, and divide—which brings me to your daughter's next important biological right.

BIOLOGICAL RIGHT #2—MAKE FRIENDS WITH FAT CELLS

This biological female right may sound more like science-fiction fantasy, but it can be a reality. You have no other option but to help your daughter befriend her fat cells. If she doesn't, she may live a life of weight preoccupation, body dissatisfaction, dieting, and disordered eating. From Chapter 3, you know the effects of dieting on fat cells—it makes them larger and more efficient in storage. So, *if you can't beat them through dieting, join them through friendship.*

Prior to puberty, a young girl's body carries only 12 percent body fat. But with the surge of estrogen at puberty, those dormant, prepubertal fat cells undergo a transformation. They start multiplying, storing, and enlarging. When enough fat has been stored to bring her body fat up to 17 percent, her body realizes that there is sufficient fat to menstruate and signals the start of her first period. But the fat cells' mission is not over yet. They keep dividing until their numbers reach 30 billion, and they keep storing until a young girl's body fat reaches 22 percent—which is about enough stored fat to survive a nine-month famine. Her fat cells are indispensable; they ensure her female status, her survival, and the survival of a developing child. Just in case she's pregnant when this anticipated famine hits, her fat cells want to make sure that she has enough reserves to carry the child to full term.

Much of the fat she gains will be in her breasts, buttocks, hips, and thighs. All women need to carry ample fat on their lower bodies to stay fertile *and* stay healthy. Being pear-shaped increases her life expectancy a full eight years (compared to men) by lowering her risk of heart disease, cancer, and diabetes. Because of fat's life-extending and life-giving properties, there was a time when being thin was considered a terrible misfortune for women, a pregnancy and health risk, and fat was considered a blessing, a sign of reproductive strength and good health. But today, female fat is erroneously viewed as a sign of character weakness and an unhealthy excess.

Inform your daughter that female fat is vital, necessary, and healthy—and alert her to an important medical fact: ***You can't fight a fat cell, and you can't pare a pear-shaped body.*** After you've shared this biological right of passage with your daughter, she may not even want to try to fight needed fat because she'll consider the female fat cell more of a friend than an enemy.

BIOLOGICAL RIGHT #3—MAKE PEACE WITH PERIODS

Just as women need to make friends with their fat cells, they also need to make peace with their periods. Once young women start their menstrual cycles, they will have 450 periods and about 6,000 potential days of premenstrual changes ahead of them. That's almost a third of their lives! And they can live life more peacefully if they understand and accept their menstrual cycles.

Here are some questions your daughter may ask about PMS and her periods along with some examples of responses.

1. **Why Do I Feel Bloated?** As hormones change after you ovulate, your body retains water (not fat!), and you may gain two to four pounds of water weight before each period. Much of that increase in water weight will be in your abdomen, breasts, face, hands, and feet. Your clothes may fit uncomfortably, your bra may be a bit tighter than usual, and your shoes and rings may feel tighter too. Your body retains water to ensure that all of your cells are properly hydrated during this special time of the month. But the two- to four-pound weight gain is not permanent! As soon as your period starts, you'll lose the water weight by urinating more frequently. In the meantime, wear looser, more comfortable clothing.

2. **Why Do I Feel Sensitive and Emotional?** After you ovulate, your changing hormones (estrogen and progesterone) affect some of the brain cells that influence your mood, energy, and spirits. This is completely normal. You may feel sad or irritable—or you may feel more alert and creative. Many artists and writers report that some of their best work was accomplished during the premenstrual days. But each month may bring different emotions, so what's most important is that you are aware of your feelings and let yourself experience them—cry, laugh, be sociable, or be private.

3. **Why Am I Craving Chocolate and Sweets?** Feeling emotional and experiencing food cravings go hand in hand. The same brain cells that influence your moods are also requesting the ingredients in chocolate and other sweets to stabilize your mood and lift your energy level. These are positive food messages; listen to them and make yourself happy! Don't worry, your brain cells don't need five candy bars (although it may seem like they do sometimes); less than half a candy bar will satisfy your craving and help make you feel better.

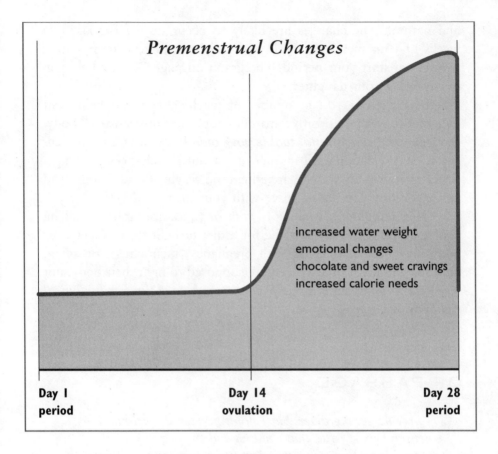

Premenstrual Changes

increased water weight
emotional changes
chocolate and sweet cravings
increased calorie needs

Day 1   **Day 14**   **Day 28**
period   **ovulation**   **period**

4. **Why Am I Hungry All the Time?** During the last two weeks of the menstrual cycle, your body needs more calories, and you'll get hungry more often. Up to an extra 150 calories are needed per day because your body is laying down the lining in your uterus and getting ready to menstruate. These extra calories will be burned up quickly and will not cause weight gain. Most mothers and daughters think that this is the best news yet about PMS. Eat more and not gain weight. Some have even done the math and figured out that 12 months × 14 premenstrual days in each month × 150 calories/day = 25,200 extra calories a year! They can't wait for their next period!

Having an increased appetite, craving chocolate, and feeling bloated and emotional are biologically based and perfectly normal

75

and natural. The changes are likely to occur during the last two weeks of your menstrual cycle and will be strongest the few days before you start your period. The graph on page 75 may help you in educating your daughter.

I have given you a number of teaching skills to help your daughter form more positive attitudes about her premenstrual body. *But your best educational tool is your own body.* If you are a menstruating, premenopausal mother, point out the changes you experience in your body weight, appetite, food cravings, and moods. And articulate how you are at peace with your menstrual cycles.

Your daughter is looking to you for validation of her changing female body. If you are looking for a diet to fight the changes your body may be experiencing with pregnancy, menopause, or aging, then she will learn that women are supposed to fight their body, not respect and appreciate it. *Help your daughter claim her biological rights by reclaiming yours.*

A MOTHER'S BIOLOGICAL RIGHT OF PASSAGE

> *I may be getting older, but I don't necessarily feel like I'm getting better. After two children and the beginnings of menopause, I've completely lost my figure despite all my dieting and exercising.*
>
> —*Martha, age 45*

Body dissatisfaction, desire for thinness, low self-esteem—the same feelings that accompany young women during puberty are also shared by their mothers during pregnancy (and after) and at menopause. Most women are not fully prepared for the body changes and believe that they can retain their youthful figure because of society's false representation of mature female passage:

- Prepregnancy weight can be achieved within six months of childbirth.
- Breast-feeding is a foolproof method of weight loss.

- Menopausal weight gain can be prevented.

- The aging process doesn't and shouldn't cause weight gain.

If we don't meet these expectations and instead gain weight, we are informed it's because we lack willpower and discipline.

Forget willpower and discipline—female physiology cannot be controlled or negotiated with. Fat cells cannot be disciplined. As a matter of fact, fat cells are working to protect you and keep you healthy—*they are on your side.*

As I continue with a woman's biological rights of passage, the fourth and fifth rights are for you to reclaim as well as to share with your daughter so that she will have a full understanding of the future of her maturing body.

BIOLOGICAL RIGHT #4—BE PREPARED FOR POSTPREGNANCY POUNDS

While pregnancy is a wonderful experience for most women, post-pregnancy turns out to be a frustrating time for almost all of us. Because estrogen is responsible for the activity of our female fat cells, the high estrogen levels during pregnancy encourage our fat cells to store up to eleven extra pounds of fat for a healthy pregnancy and delivery. More fat storage enzymes are stimulated, and more fat cells are formed. Pregnancy, like puberty, is a time in a woman's life when fat storage is so important that fat cells divide to make sure plenty of room is available for storage. And, knowing the stubborn nature of fat cells, once they store fat, they want to lock it up and throw away the key. That's why those last five to ten pounds of pregnancy weight are the most difficult to lose.[6]

Along with the extra stubborn fat come some other "extras" that women need to prepare for: extra hip width, extra waist inches, and extra skin on the stomach. How prepared are or were you for these changes?

"Nobody really told me what would happen to my body," one new mother shared. "Some magazine articles I read said that I could get back into my prepregnancy jeans within six weeks if I exercised and followed their plan. My nurses and doctors promised me that I would lose weight quicker if I breast-fed. What they didn't tell me was that they were only trying to make me feel better. Instead, my hipbones separated—permanently—and breast-feeding kept my appetite up and my fat cells active. I ran into an old friend six weeks after delivery and she asked me when the baby was due. I was devastated."

The reality is: postpregnancy weight-loss plans don't fulfill their promises and breast-feeding may not guarantee weight loss.[7] Breast-feeding has many wonderful benefits for both infant and mother, including contraction of the uterus, which brings it and other organs back into place. But, during lactation, hormone levels are still high, and fat cells want to hold on to their stored fat to provide a reserve of calories just in case that pending famine hits. As a matter of fact, some women's fat cells won't give up much fat until *after* they've stopped breast-feeding.

Several health professionals I have spoken with are fearful of informing women that breast-feeding is not a foolproof method to shed pregnancy pounds. One said, "If I tell my patients that some women don't lose weight quickly while breast-feeding, they may opt for the bottle over the breast." I understand this physician's concern, but my own experience with clients has differed from this "my body's more important than my baby" attitude. Instead, my clients have appreciated my honesty, chosen to breast-feed for its multitude of benefits, and have had realistic expectations of their bodies after pregnancy.

You are a source of information for your daughter—and you are also a role model during this time. If you are pregnant or have recently delivered your second (or third or fourth) child, and you have a young daughter, she is going to witness and absorb your reaction to your changing body. Pregnancy can be a time in our lives to come to terms with the authenticity of the female body and to stop being obsessed with being thin. As one woman said, "I loved being pregnant, watching my stomach grow and feeling the baby move. I was always the type who fasted for a day if I gained a pound, so I can't believe I'm saying this—but so what if I have a few extra pounds and wider hips; I have a healthy child and a strong body."

If, instead, your reaction is one of preoccupation, self-consciousness, or anger, your daughter may develop negative feelings toward pregnancy and her own body. This happened to fifteen-year-old Megan, whose excessive dieting had caused her reproductive system to shut down. I was counseling her to increase her food intake and body fat so that she would start menstruating again and improve her chances of fertility later on in life. But menstruation and fertility were not motivating goals for her. "I don't care if I never start my period again because I don't want to have children. I've seen my mother's agony with her body after childbirth, and she blames me and my two younger brothers for her weight struggles. I certainly don't want to go through that if I don't have to."

For your daughter as well as for yourself, accepting how your body changes during pregnancy and understanding why some of the changes may be permanent are pivotal behaviors. If you are not able to accept these changes, you may embark on the disordered eating path and take your daughter along it with you. In fact, postpregnancy has recently been identified as one of the two new high-risk times for developing eating disorders. The other time is during the transition to menopause.

BIOLOGICAL RIGHT #5—BE MINDFUL OF THE MENOPAUSAL WEIGHT GAIN

Over the next twenty years, as more baby boomers reach middle age, an estimated 40 million women will enter menopause, and the nation may experience a simultaneous hot flash (or power surge, as some call it). Accompanying that massive surge of body heat will be a dramatic drop in body happiness as millions of women cry out for help with their expanding waistlines and midlife weight crises.

As with puberty and postpregnancy, that cry for help can be answered through education and understanding of the healthy passage through menopause: the third and final stage in a woman's life when a change in fat cell physiology and body shape occurs.

As estrogen levels are dropping and women are winding down their menstrual cycles, you would think that fat cells would become less active because they are no longer needed for fertility, pregnancy, and breast-feeding. But a woman's fat cells are smarter than that—they find other ways to stay active and other reasons to keep storing fat.

During the transition to menopause, metabolism can decrease 15 to 20 percent, which means that the body's calorie needs are lower. Because we're eating the same amount of food, the fat cells have more left over to store. In addition, as estrogen levels drop, the male sex hormone, testosterone (always present in a woman's body in small amounts), starts to have a greater influence and activates the fat cells in the abdominal area. Because of testosterone, when men gain weight, it's almost always in the abdominal area. Therefore, when menopausal women gain weight, it's also more likely to be in the waist. That's why skirts and pants still fit everywhere else but are often too tight in the waist.

The combination of a slower metabolism and the stimulation of abdominal fat cells can result in an eight- to twelve-pound weight gain for many women. Can you prevent it? Somewhat, but not entirely. Exercise boosts metabolism and is the most effective way to deter fat gain. One study showed that menopausal women who exercised regularly gained one-half of the body fat of those who did not exercise.[8] But they still gained some stubborn fat because menopausal women need some extra fat for four important reasons:

1. Fat is the primary source of estrogen production for postmenopausal women. As the ovaries and the adrenal gland stop producing estrogen, the fat cells take over some of the responsibility. The body knows that the more fat it stores, the more estrogen it will produce.

2. The estrogen produced by the fat cells helps to lessen the symptoms of menopause. This explains why underweight women report significantly more menopausal symptoms, and overweight women report fewer hot flashes, mood changes, and sleep difficulties. Fat cells are looking out for our well-being.

3. The extra weight gained helps to reduce the risk of osteoporosis and hip fractures because as the bones carry around that additional weight every day, they become stronger.

4. Gaining a few extra pounds during midlife may decrease mortality later on in life. Underweight seniors are more likely to die younger because they lack the reserves to withstand illness. But those who

gain a moderate amount of weight with age live longer.[9] (If you are thinking about the recent, well-publicized Harvard study showing that women who were 15 percent below their recommended weight lived the longest, the media failed to report on the whole story and the study failed to control for a number of factors.[10])

After hearing these compelling reasons for menopausal weight gain, most of my clients look as if they had twenty pounds of anxiety lifted from them. Fewer menopausal symptoms, stronger bones, and a longer life sound pretty good to them. *Fat cells really are concerned with our well-being!*

The combination of pubertal changes, pregnancy weight gain(s), and menopausal weight gain explains why women are more likely to experience greater weight gain throughout life than men. Weight gain peaks for men at age forty-four; for women, at age fifty-five, after the transition to menopause. And between the ages of twenty-five and fifty-five, women gain an average of sixteen pounds from the combination of pregnancies, menopause, and aging.[11]

If men had an abundance of estrogen instead of testosterone and underwent the physiological changes of the menstrual cycle and menopause, they too would carry more fat and gain more weight throughout life. But as long as most men exercise regularly and have reasonable eating habits, they can maintain a leaner figure. As one perturbed client pointed out, "My husband hasn't gained an ounce since the day I met him twenty years ago. The differences between men and women are hard enough to understand, but why do our two most unique life cycles, *men*arche and *men*opause, have the word 'men' in them? I bet men label these terms to stroke their egos." Although I found my client's observation interesting, the truth is, "men" is a Greek derivative meaning "month," so menarche means the beginning of monthly blood flow and menopause means the end of monthly blood flow.

Before leaving this discussion of a mother's biological rights of passage, a recent phenomenon deserves mention. More and more women are choosing to have children in the latter part of their childbearing years and then shortly thereafter entering the transition to menopause. Although this phenomenon has not yet been researched, my observation with over 100 clients is that these women's bodies are unable to lose the weight gained during pregnancy before an additional layer of fat is deposited with menopause. And thus, their frustration and preoccupation with weight intensifies.

This frustration is important to address because these mothers will be at odds with the ten- to fifteen-year transition to menopause at the same time their daughters are fighting the transition to puberty. When I shared this phenomenon with one menopausal mother, she quickly noted the similarities between her and her adolescent daughter. "Both of our moods are swinging like a pendulum, and both of our bodies are storing fat like bears preparing for hibernation." If you find this to be the case for you and your daughter, use it as an opportunity to work closely together to accept your body changes.

Thus far, what I have shared with you regarding the healthy biological passage holds true for all women. Each of us has estrogen, but each of us also has or will have a unique, slightly different experience through each phase. Some young women lay down more fat in their hips during puberty; others more in their thighs. Some women gain fifteen pounds with pregnancy; others gain fifty plus. Some women gain twenty pounds during the transition of menopause; others gain two. Some women are genetically predisposed to be overweight; others are genetically programmed to be underweight. How you and your daughter journey through each passage of womanhood is determined, to a large extent, by genetics.

ACCEPTING GENETIC ENDOWMENT

It took me thirty years to realize that my thunder thighs came from a long line of strong female genes. My grandmother had them, my mother has them, my sister and I have them—and no doubt my daughter will have them too. I had best share with her the lightning bolt reality of thunder thighs in the McKinley family.

—Julie, age 34

We all need to reflect on genetic influences in our lives and share these observations with our daughters. Genetics can and does make a difference in how our body matures and takes shape, how it responds to pregnancy and menopause, and how it gains and loses weight.

Just as we are born with a genetically predetermined foot size that we must accept, we are also born with a predetermined bone structure, frame size, and body shape that we must accept. And, most likely, your body's genetic blueprint came from your mother and your daughter's will come from you.

How similar is your body to your mother's when she was your age? How much weight did your mother gain during pregnancy? How does your weight gain compare? If you look at your mother's body and find no similarities, look to your grandmother. Genetic influences sometimes skip a generation.

Many of my clients are amazed when they spend a moment thinking of the similarities between their bodies and their mothers':

- "I could put my head on my mother's body and you wouldn't be able to tell us apart."

- "My mother gained 44 pounds during pregnancy, and I gained exactly 44 pounds."

- "My mother weighs 168 pounds and I weighed 166 pounds—until I got off my butt and started exercising."

- "My mother has been obese since childhood, and so have I."

What about the genetic influence on obesity? This is where heredity becomes more of a gray area. Some studies, such as those of the Pima Indians, a tribe that has one of the highest incidences of obesity, have shown that obesity tendencies are passed directly from the mother to the daughter.[12] Other studies have shown that lifestyle accounts for 75 percent of the overall cause of obesity while genetics accounts for only 25 percent.[13] The University of Illinois concluded that "genetics may predispose an individual toward obesity, but family environment, particularly child feeding practices and other environmental variables . . . serve as a catalyst for the expression of obesity."[14] So, if an obesity gene does lurk in your family tree, an environment of disordered eating and a sedentary lifestyle activate it.

Frame size, bone structure, body shape, and, in some cases, obesity are genetically predetermined and usually passed from the mother to the daughter. However, for some daughters, the stronger genetic link may be with their fathers or grandfathers. In either case, use your family history and genetic endowment to understand the origins of your and your daughter's body shape—and use your lifestyle habits to understand why you and/or your daughter may be carrying more weight than is healthy.

In my first counseling session with a client, I ask, "Why do you think you are carrying extra weight?" I can't begin to count the number of women who answer "Because my mother is overweight. I inherited her body, and I am doomed by genetics." Most daughters are not genetically doomed to be fat, but they are genetically endowed with a certain body structure and shape that they can affect either positively or negatively with their own behavior and lifestyle choices. Keep in mind that all women are genetically and physiologically linked by their larger fat cells and pear-shaped bodies. Oftentimes it may appear that the mother has willed a fatter body to the daughter—but that's mother nature's fault, not mother's.

We need to accept both our gender and our genetics. Show your young daughter a picture of yourself during your own teen years so that she will have a vision of what her body may look like. If the women in your family characteristically have large thighs, let your daughter know that lifestyle changes through exercise and eating habits will not produce thin thighs. But they will result in smaller thighs.

If you are an overweight mother, genetically or otherwise, and carry the extra burden that your weight may be the cause of your daughter's poor body image and disordered eating, lighten your load. Practically every study has shown that a mother's weight isn't a determining factor. Rather it is the mother's attitudes about her weight and her behaviors around food that correlate with how the daughter forms her body image and structures her own eating behavior. Genetically underweight mothers who are weight preoccupied can pass on negative body images to their daughters, and genetically overweight mothers who are at peace with their bodies can endow their daughters with positive body images.

In our thin-worshipping society, is it possible to be overweight *and* like your body? As organizations such as the National Association to Advance Fat Acceptance (NAAFA) and Women Insisting On Natural Shapes (WINS) continue to help women with body acceptance, it is definitely possible. One group of women has proven it with little, if any, outside assistance: the African American female community. They are more likely to be overweight, but they are also more likely to have an accepting attitude and a healthy passage through womanhood regardless of their weight.

APPRECIATING ETHNIC HERITAGE

My mother is overweight, but she is a beautiful, strong,
black woman. I have her body, and that's okay because it
means that I'm beautiful and strong too.
—Clarissa, age 13

Of all ethnic groups, African American women have the highest incidence of obesity: 49.2 percent are overweight.[15] Yet despite the higher prevalence of obesity, 40 percent of those who are overweight still view their bodies as attractive, and almost 100 percent of them report no negative effects from being overweight on their personal or family relationships.[16] How many Caucasian mothers can say the same is true of their lives?

For African American women, the phrase "like mother, like daughter" means a generational transfer of body acceptance. Almost half of the overweight black daughters report that they are satisfied with their appearance,[17] and at all weights, black female adolescents are seven times more likely to be content with their bodies than white adolescents.[18] Happiness with their bodies equates with higher self-esteem even during the turbulent teen years. The AAUW study found that between the ages of nine and fifteen, black female adolescents' self-esteem dropped only 7 percentage points while whites' dropped 33 percentage points.[19]

As would be expected, the more positive the body image and the higher the self-esteem, the more unlikely it is that both mother and daughter will become active participants in the dieting game.

Almost all of the white daughters I interviewed reported that their mothers had dieted, but few of the black daughters remembered their mothers dieting. To the question: "Did your mother diet?" one daughter responded, "Diet!! She had more important things to do. She was a single mother of four kids and worked full-time. She always told us that 'black was beautiful' and loved her body just the way it was."

Why is the ethnic influence so positive for the African American female community? Researchers believe the reason primarily lies in the strong, communicative mother-daughter relationship where mothers are viewed as powerful role models and wise, beautiful matriarchs. In fact, the majority of young black girls rated their mothers as currently beautiful whereas the majority of young white girls reported that their mothers were once beautiful in their younger years.[20]

For the black female community, the definition of beauty goes far beyond thinness. While adult white women have to weigh a low 117 pounds to feel attractive, adult black women can weigh 145 pounds and still feel good about their bodies.[21] And this strong body acceptance continues into the senior years. In a study that compared black and white women ages 66 to 102, the African American seniors were three times more likely to find themselves attractive even though they were twice as likely to be obese.[22] No wonder black adolescent girls have more positive body images; both their mothers *and* grandmothers model body acceptance.

Not only do African American women accept having larger bodies, they also seem to know instinctively what are their realistic physical limits of weight loss. This instinct was apparent with one young black woman's brief flirtation with dieting. "I went to join Nutrisystem once, but they told me that I needed to lose thirty-five pounds to reach my 'ideal' weight according to their charts. I burst into laughter and walked out. My body would *never* lose that much weight." Physically, black women carry more muscle mass (which weighs more than fat) and have a denser bone structure, so they are more likely to be larger and to be labeled overweight when they get on the scale at a weight-loss clinic or doctor's office.

However, not all black women have such body wisdom and acceptance. As American lifestyles have become more homogeneous and women of all colors have fallen victim to the same ideal body image, for the first time in history disordered eating and eating disorders have crossed race and economic barriers. But their incidence in the black community is still below their occurrence in the white, middle-class world.[23]

The black female community has been extensively studied for the overwhelmingly positive effects of ethnic heritage on body acceptance. But for other ethnic groups, far less research is available. American Indian and Hispanic women also have high incidences of obesity,[24] but they do not share the body acceptance of the African American female community. Studies show that American Indian[25] and Hispanic[26] women are more similar to whites in their body dissatisfaction, body perceptions, and dieting practices.

From the scant studies on Asian women, it appears that they are less likely to diet than any other ethnic group.[27] Why? Genetically they carry leaner and smaller bodies, and socially they were never conditioned to start dieting because dieting goes against their eating philosophy. One of the Japanese dietary guidelines (which I wish were one of ours) is "to make all activities pertaining to food and eating pleasurable ones."[28] I can think of many words to describe dieting, but pleasurable is *not* one of them.

There is much to learn from the Asian and black female communities: Asian women can teach us that dieting is philosophically undesirable, and black women can teach us that a variety of body shapes and sizes is socially desirable. In addition, mothers and daughters of all races can join together to accept the healthy biological passage through womanhood and initiate a revolutionary change in the way women perceive their bodies, a shift that will resonate through contemporary culture and free women from the thin ideal.

CHAPTER FIVE

ONE SIZE DOES NOT FIT ALL: THE MOTHER–DAUGHTER BODY REVOLUTION

Sara is lying on the couch thumbing through a teen magazine when she spots what she is looking for: a model who has the exact body she so desperately wants. As she tears out the page, her mind drifts back to her best friend boasting about her new size-2 jeans at school that day, her boyfriend commenting on how great her friend looked, and her track coach recommending that she lose at least another five pounds before the first meet. She glances at the television and her favorite show, *Beverly Hills 90210,* is about to start. She carefully studies Tori Spelling's and Jennie Garth's thin bodies and daydreams about how exciting life would be if only she were thin.

In one day, fifteen-year-old Sara is exposed to five different sources of pressure to lose weight and achieve the thin ideal: magazine models, her peers, her boyfriend, her coach, and television celebrities. Each and every day, Sara and millions of other teenagers are comparing themselves to an unattainable representation of the female body and resorting to unhealthy behaviors to pursue this unhealthy ideal.

Do you remember how old you were when you first discovered that your body didn't measure up to the supposed ideal? Who was your first symbol of the ideal female body? One mother answered, "I was sixteen, and I wanted to be Farrah Fawcett. I wanted her body, hair, smile—the whole package. I tried for ten years, then gave up and have hated my body ever since."

Whoever you may have idealized, through years of experience you now probably understand that trying to match the ideal is biologically impossible and psychologically damaging. By sharing these important realizations with your daughter, you may be able to prevent her from spending most of her childhood and adolescence unhappy with her body and preoccupied with her weight. She needs your wisdom. As the images of young female celebrities infiltrate the subconscious minds of girls at ever younger ages, the petite measurements of Kate Moss and Tori Spelling serve as a goal for far too many. This early awareness of thinness causes poor body images in the majority of girls in every age group studied.

You can have an important role in formulating a more realistic representation of female identity by helping your daughter put these media images in perspective. Even if you place no pressure on your daughter to conform to a thin ideal, as soon as she walks out the door, turns on the television, or opens a magazine, the pressure to be thin is in full force. In one issue of *Seventeen* magazine, I found sixty-two photographs of unnaturally thin models accompanying articles and advertisements. In three hours of network prime-time television, the images of twenty-seven slender females conveyed the unspoken message that thinness brings happiness, popularity, and male attention. In one hour of MTV programming, thirty-three different women displayed their slim bodies on music videos. As the primary source of the impossible ideal, these media images play a predominant role in the shaping, or rather the unshaping, of our daughters' female identity. Challenging the power of the media's influence may seem overwhelming, but you can have a positive influence on your daughter's body image and self-esteem by empathizing with her feelings, encouraging her to appreciate her own physique, and deemphasizing beauty messages.

RE-VIEW YOUR BODY IMAGE

*Both my daughter and I make degrading comments about
our bodies every day. How can we upgrade our body
image?*

—Kim, age 41

All mothers I have spoken with are eager to help themselves and to
make a difference in their daughters' lives. I'm sure that you are too.
To begin, you need to know where you and your daughter stand on
your own body images. In other words, how does the picture in
your mind of how you think you should look compare with how
you actually look? For most of us, that dreamlike image is unrealistic
and causes us to judge ourselves harshly. Simply asking the question
"Do you like your body?" does not always elicit an accurate response. We may know that we don't like our bodies, but we do not
know the extent of our dissatisfaction or the negative impact it's
having on our lives.

Assessment questionnaires can be helpful tools. Answer "yes"
or "no" to the following ten questions to determine where you stand
on body image and self-esteem, then have your daughter answer
these same questions. I recommend covering up your own answers
so they don't bias your daughter's.

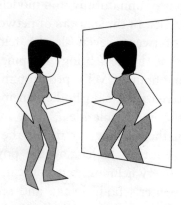

Do You Need to Work as a Team to Build Body Image and Self-Esteem?

	YOU	YOUR DAUGHTER
1. Do you weigh yourself daily?		
2. If you were thinner, do you think you'd be happier?		
3. Does your weight determine how you feel about yourself?		
4. Do you compare your body to other women's?		
5. Do you feel depressed when looking through fashion magazines?		
6. Do you feel self-conscious around thinner women?		
7. Is clothes shopping a dreaded activity?		
8. Do you hide your body in loose clothing?		
9. Do you avoid social events because of your weight?		
10. Do you blame your weight struggles on genetics?		
TOTAL # OF "YES" ANSWERS		

If you and/or your daughter answered "yes" to seven to ten of these questions, then YES! it's time to work as a team to build body image and self-esteem. If you had three to six "yes" responses, then you also need to work together, but you may have already begun to befriend your body. If you had fewer than three "yes" answers (given our society, a zero score is unrealistic), then you have an accepting, accurate body image—regardless of what you weigh. Was it because your mother advocated body acceptance? Was it because you long ago decided to let go of society's pressure for thinness?

Also, compare your and your daughter's answers. More likely

than not, they are similar. The phrase "like mother, like daughter" holds true for dieting practices, disordered eating behaviors—and body image.

Now, irrespective of your scores, the most important question is: *What can you do today to start befriending your body and to help your daughter befriend hers?*

Having counseled thousands of women over the years, I will share some of the strategies that have been most helpful for my clients—as well as for myself. Unlike many books on body image, my advice is not to "fix" or "change" or "better" your body from the outside; it's to feel good about yourself from the *inside*.

Focusing only on improving our looks is futile because there is little connection between actual physical attractiveness and body image and self-esteem. That's why losing weight or undergoing cosmetic surgery does not necessarily correlate with improved body image and self-esteem. We are told that makeovers and makeup will make us feel better about ourselves—but that's make-believe. So, we spend about $50 billion a year on cosmetics, plastic surgery, and dieting without much improvement in body image or self-esteem. As Peggy Ornstein so accurately wrote in her eye-opening book *School Girls*, "How terribly clever, . . . the people who robbed women of their self-esteem now want to sell it back to us!"[1]

Instead of trying to "buy" a positive body image, you can discover that you already have one; it's just buried beneath false expectations, unrealistic cultural ideals, and a misunderstanding of the female body. The suggestions in this chapter will help you to uncover your and your daughter's positive, more accepting body image. The best place to start is with society's impossible ideal.

SOCIETY'S JEANS vs. BIOLOGICAL GENES: AN IMPOSSIBLE FIT

*I'm down to 103 pounds but my thighs are still too big
and my hipbones still don't stick out enough.*
                                        —*Penelope, age 11*

Thin thighs and protruding hipbones are foremost on the minds of young girls. Add perfectly flat stomachs, visible rib cages, boney upper arms, and very little body fat—and we have their version of the ideal body: one that looks as if it hasn't been fed in over a month. Unfortunately, most young fashion models today look like this.

Standing at 5 foot 10½ inches tall and weighing 114 pounds, the typical model displays the visible signs of chronic starvation. In contrast, the typical American woman stands at 5 foot 4½ inches tall and weighs 140 pounds. Real women and the unreal ideal are many pounds, inches, and sizes apart.

	UNREAL IDEAL	REAL WOMAN
HEIGHT	70½"	64½"
WEIGHT	114 lbs.	140 lbs.
BODY FAT	10–15%	22–32%
CLOTHING SIZE	4–6	12–14

We would have to stretch our bodies by six inches, drop half of our body fat, shrink four clothing sizes, and lose almost 25 percent of our body weight to mold our bodies to the present female ideal body. *An undeniable biological impossibility!*

But not only are we dissatisfied with our bodies because we weigh 25 percent more than the ideal, we also see ourselves as larger than we actually are. The University of Florida found that 95 percent of the underweight, normal-weight, and overweight women studied overestimated their body size by 25 percent![2] So, not only do we weigh 25 percent more than the ideal, we also magnify our body size by another 25 percent. No wonder we are weight preoccupied and have negative body images—many of us see ourselves as being *50 percent* away from the undernourished ideal.

Overestimation of body size—the amount of space we take up and what we see in the mirror—is common to women of all ages. I've counseled women who erroneously believe that they can't fit into airline seats or restaurant booths, and I've counseled young girls who inaccurately choose clothing sizes that are two sizes too big.

The ideal may be unrealistic for most women, but the body size distortions and negative feelings it provokes are very real. One client described her body dissatisfaction as "something that definitely hinders me, but my kids are my top priority so they keep my mind occupied," while another client shared her obsessive "bad body" thoughts as "the only thing that holds me back, keeps me from having children, getting a satisfying job, and working on my relationship with my husband." I have come across thousands of women who put their lives on hold until they lost weight, only to realize one day that they spent the last ten or twenty or thirty years not living. I know a creative advertising executive who sometimes stayed home from work because she felt fat. I know another successful business owner who found excuses to avoid business trips because she feared the minibar in her hotel room. I know a gifted college professor who was forced to take sabbatical because her exercise addiction became more important than her students' education. All of these gifted, creative women were obsessed with trying to achieve society's impossible ideal. Are you?

Unless you and your daughter are among the small minority born with the bone structure, height, metabolism, and body composition to coincide with today's unreal ideal, nothing short of a miracle will transform your body to its dimensions. But nonetheless, we try. And if at first we don't succeed, we try, try again. We diet, skip meals, fast, take diet pills and fat-burning pills, and exercise three hours a day. Then we conclude that we are inferior, inadequate, and less of a woman. But most of us fail to recognize the irony in our conclusion. *The emaciated ideal is literally less of a woman—not us.*

This discussion of our culture's unrealistic female icons would not be complete without commenting on Barbie. As a journalist pointed out in a recent issue of *Self* magazine, unrealistic is an understatement! This writer produced the following calculations to show how much her body would have to change to coincide with Barbie's proportions: her bust would have to expand twelve inches, her waist would have to shrink ten inches, and she would have to grow to be a towering seven feet two inches tall.[3] Unfortunately, Barbie is often a young girl's first exposure to the unhealthy ideal—and the doll's popularity continues to grow.

Some mothers' initial reaction to Barbie's popularity is to forbid their daughters to play with the doll. But boycotting may only increase a girl's fascination. Instead, let her interest pass and in the meantime use Barbie as an educational tool, describing the differences between her plastic body and those of living, breathing women. One of my favorite descriptions of Barbie is by Oni Faida Lampley, an African American playwright, who wrote, "What a sweet toy for a little black girl, a rubber-headed, relentlessly white woman with plastic torpedo titties, no hips, no ass, who needed a kickstand up her butt to stand because she was permanently poised on the balls of her feet."[4]

Whether it's dolls, fashion models, film stars, or television celebrities, the petite figures many of them exhibit are the exception. Remind yourself of this important fact and teach your daughter how unreal the thin ideal is by comparing the average model with the typical woman. In addition, share with your daughter another blunt reality: picture-perfect models are less than perfect. They do not crawl out of bed looking like the image in the glossy photo. Expert makeup artists provide the perfect coloring, hairstylists add body and shine, and skilled photographers take hundreds of photographs with perfect lighting, angles, and shadows. Then, after the best photo is chosen, up to four hours of retouching begins to eliminate any evidence of pores, lines, or imperfections. At times, the head of one model may be used on the body of another. Today, with computer technology, the possibilities are endless. The beauty ideal has always been unreal, but now when we look at pictures, we don't even know what's simulated and what isn't.

Another effective suggestion is to take a magazine picture of a model that your daughter idolizes, go to the mall or grocery store, and have your daughter search for someone who has a similar body. She may be there for hours and eventually conclude that the beautiful, thin, flawless image in the photo is indeed a myth.

The need to dispel the many beauty myths is more urgent than ever. In one of my attempts to meet that need, I was a guest lecturer in a middle-school biology class. I encourage you to use the same or a similar teaching technique with your daughter as I used with this class. I had the students write down their responses to the question: If you could change your body with a blink of an eye, what would be different? Then, to open discussion, I randomly chose one student's response:

> I would be ten pounds lighter, wear a size four, have no fat on my body whatsoever, have thighs the size of my upper arms with no cellulite, have hipbones that stick out, and have ribs that stick out. I guess the only thing I would keep would be my head, but I would be a natural blonde.

My discussion started with the easiest myth to dispel: *the blond myth.* I asked the class, "Who wants to be a blonde? and if you do, why?" Most of the nonblond girls raised their hands, reasoning that "blondes are prettier and more popular" or "blondes have more fun." I don't know of any study that investigated whether blondes have more fun or not, but when I shared the results of a study that revealed blondes have the lowest level of self-confidence, the young women were surprised. Redheads have the highest level of self-confidence, followed by brunettes; last on the list is blondes.[5] The redheads immediately sat up straighter.

Next, I attacked *the protruding hipbone myth.* I showed a transparency of the female abdominal organs, where they are located, and how their natural roundness needs to be cushioned by some fat. Then I explained that in order for the hipbones to stick out, most women would either have to be in a state of chronic starvation or have their internal organs removed. The class was visibly disturbed when I told them about a women who went to the extreme of having a hysterectomy in hopes that the removal of her uterus and ovaries would flatten her stomach.

I saved *the thin thigh myth* for last. The thighs are the number-one disliked body part for women young and old, and adolescent girls are almost twice as likely to dislike their thighs as any other body part.[6] Although they were disappointed to hear that fat-free thighs were a biological impossibility, the class understood the physiological explanation for ample fat on a woman's thighs. The area where the thighs attach to the buttocks and hips has the most concentrated number of fat cells—and the most stubborn fat cells because it's the most important area for female fertility. The young women were also disappointed to hear that cellulite-free thighs were equally impossible. Cellulite may look different, but it's just another name for fat—a marketing term instead of a medical term. Some of the young women in the class had tried cellulite lotions and potions and appreciated my alternative definition of cellulite—"sell-you-lie-t"—because those who promote these products are selling you nothing less than a lie. Cellulite cannot be dissolved or disintegrated; it can only be disguised temporarily with products that tighten the skin or plump up the tissue. But any perceived change is a short-lived illusion. The only long-term solution is to reduce body fat through exercise.

Toward the end of the class, one student raised her hand and shared her confusion. "By your definition, I'm a perfectly healthy, developing woman, but by my doctor's definition, I'm overweight and need to lose eleven pounds."

As unrealistic and unhealthy as the ideal promoted by the media may be, the health industry continues to give it credence. The message from the fashion industry is "be thin to be happy"; the message from the health industry is "be thin to be healthy." The media has always promised happiness with a thin body, but beware as it capitalizes on the health promises of weight loss and a thin body. In July 1995, I did an analysis of weight-loss articles in thirty-seven magazines. All of the women's magazines had at least one weight-loss article; some had as many as four, with cover lines such as "Drop a Dress Size in Two Weeks" and "Drop 10 Pounds in 10 Days"—but overall, over half of the articles approached thinness and weight loss from a health angle. After all, it's unhealthy to be overweight—or is it?

FIND COMFORT IN YOUR BODY'S HEALTHY WEIGHT

*My body may not be accepted by society, but it's the only
one I have. It's fit, strong, and dependable.*
—Heather, age 38

I suppose the first question to answer is: What is a healthy weight? Let
me begin answering this question by first telling you what it isn't:

- It is *not* what the height/weight charts say you should weigh. These
  charts are undergoing their seventh revision and have been all over
  the map in their weight recommendations.[7]

- It is *not* what an equation says you should weigh. A number of different equations use your height and/or age to determine your recommended weight, but they usually don't come close.

- It is *not* what Kate Moss or other models define as a "normal"
  weight. In today's culture of thinness, "normal" no longer means
  normal; it means underweight.

As you can tell, I am not a proponent of specific weight recommendations, preassigned weights, the scale, or height/weight
charts. Another weight measurement that is now widely used is BMI
(or body mass index). To calculate BMI, you must convert your
weight and height to the metric system, then do a complicated math-
ematical equation. Although BMI may be slightly more accurate
than height/weight charts, I am not an advocate of this measurement
either because you are still reduced to a number and compared to a
norm that may not apply.

We are each biologically unique; therefore, we each have a different weight that is most optimal and comfortable for us. Your
doctor, your scale, or your aerobics instructor can't tell you what
you should weigh—nobody can because only your body knows for
sure. Initially this your-body-knows-best philosophy frustrates most
of my clients. They ask, "How will I know when my body knows?
What if my body wants to be at 150 pounds?" If you are exercising
and fueling your body with positive eating habits, and your body

gravitates to a certain weight—and feels comfortable there—then that's your comfortable, healthy weight. Trying to fight it will only cause more weight gain.

How much weight you can realistically lose and where your weight will naturally stabilize is determined by your set point—the range of weight that is physiologically and psychologically optimal for your body. You're probably familiar with the set-point theory, and recently researchers at Rockefeller University have proven it.[8] When people tried to lose weight by cutting calories, their metabolisms slowed down so that they would burn less, store more, and gain the weight back. When people tried to gain weight by increasing calories, their metabolisms sped up so that they would store less, burn more, and lose the weight they gained. In other words, whenever you gain or lose weight, your body will automatically adjust its metabolism and caloric needs to keep you within your set-point range. No chart, scale, or gadget can determine your set point—only your body can determine where it feels best.

One external measurement that does come close to defining your healthy weight is percent body fat analysis because it gives you the most accurate assessment of what's happening *inside* your body. Here are the healthy body fat ranges I use that take into consideration the natural increases in body fat during puberty, pregnancy, and menopause.

HEALTHY PERCENT BODY FAT RANGES IN FEMALES

preadolescent	10 to 14%
teenager	18 to 22%
adult prepregnancy	18 to 25%
adult postpregnancy	22 to 25%
menopausal	25 to 28%

But keep in mind: *the best measurement is how your body feels, functions, and moves.*

Your healthy, comfortable weight takes into consideration genetics, where you are in the stages of female passage, your percent body fat, and your set point. These are extremely personalized variables that don't necessarily fit into charts or formulas. But the following questions will help you and your daughter determine if you are at your healthy, comfortable weight:

- Can you move freely?
- Can you exercise without huffing and puffing? (If you don't exercise and therefore can't answer this question, then you're probably not at your healthy weight.)
- Do you feel healthy?
- Are you free of weight-related problems such as high blood pressure or high blood cholesterol?
- At the end of the day, do your feet and joints feel as if they could continue carrying your body weight without discomfort (or do they feel as if they couldn't move another ounce before collapsing)?

If you answered "yes" to all these questions, no matter what you weigh, you are at a weight that is healthy for *you.*

Once you have determined whether you and your daughter are at your healthy weights, the next step is to *find comfort in that healthy weight.* The following suggestions will help you to help your daughter find comfort in her body (as well as help you find comfort in yours).

1. **Teach your daughter about her foundation.** The four important components that give her body form and allow it to function:

   - Her **bones,** which provide the basic structure of her body
   - Her **muscles,** which attach to her bones and provide the strength to stand, walk, run, rollerblade, dance, and hike
   - Her **organs,** which are necessary for breathing, thinking, digestion, and elimination of waste
   - Her **body fat,** which coats her nerve and brain cells, cushions her organs, and provides the energy for pregnancy and breast-feeding

2. **Help your daughter accept her natural pear-shaped body.** Explain the need for all women to carry extra fat on their buttocks, hips,

and thighs; share the longevity benefits of being pear-shaped and discuss how, despite weight loss, she'll still be pear-shaped.

3. **Help your daughter feel comfortable taking up space and commanding the space around her.** As you are out together, point out how body confidence is independent of weight—how some thinner women appear self-conscious and some larger women portray self-assurance.

4. **Give up the scale!** It's impossible to find comfort in our bodies when we are getting on the scale and relying on an external evaluation of self-worth.

SCALES ARE FOR FISH, NOT WOMEN

I've owned my bathroom scale for fifteen years, and that's fifteen years too long!

—Fran, age 41

Do you own a scale? How long have you had it? How often to you get on it? How does it make you feel?

- "I have one of those real doctor's scales that cost hundreds of dollars. I've tried to get rid of it, but I can't bring myself to throw away that much money."

- "I have four scales in my house—one in each bathroom, one in the bedroom, and one in the kitchen—all strategically placed so that I'm constantly reminded of my weight."

- "I keep a scale in the trunk of my car so that I can weigh myself whenever I need to. I've been known to pull over on the freeway for a curbside weigh-in."

- "I've devised a formula with my scale: If I'm up a pound, I skip one meal that day; if I'm up two pounds, I skip two meals, and so on."

- "I have one of those scales that talks to me. 'Good morning,' it says in a sickeningly cheery voice. 'You weigh 153 pounds today.' My response back is usually 'Oh, shut up (with a number of expletives)! What's so good about it? You just told me I'm fat and worthless.' "

Whether your scale talks to you or not, it does dictate how we feel about ourselves, determines what we will and will not eat that day, and decides what we will and will not wear that day. How can an inanimate, mechanical device have so much power over us?

It does because we allow the scale to be our primary measure of diet success and self-worth. But the numbers on the scale are less reliable than you think. If you get on ten different scales, you'll have ten different weights. If you get on the same scale ten different times throughout the day, you'll have ten different weights.

Try it tomorrow. Pack up your scale and take it with you. Weigh yourself ten times throughout the day and plot your weights on a graph. I'll bet you'll be as surprised as one of my clients, Carmen, was when she plotted her daily weight changes:

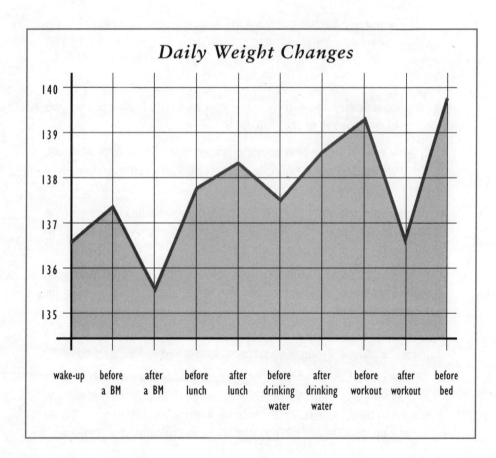

Her weight fluctuated four pounds throughout the day. It was lowest after a bowel movement and exercising (from a loss of water weight in perspiration) and highest after eating or drinking and before bed. Your weight may fluctuate as much as six pounds a day, and as the day goes on, you'll inevitably weigh more as your cells become more hydrated.

Other factors can also influence your daily weights: where you are in your menstrual cycle, the outside humidity (the higher the humidity, the higher your weight), how much salt you've eaten that day, and how much muscle mass you've developed through an exercise program. Muscle weighs more than fat, and it's not unusual to have the numbers on the scale creep up as your body is actually getting smaller.

The numbers on the scale are unreliable and constantly changing throughout the day—but do you change? No, you are the same person. That three-digit number is just a number—it is not who you are. The scale is just a mechanical device, not the determiner of whether you leave the house with a smile or a frown.

I realize that it may feel good when you get on the scale and find that it is down two or three pounds, but why do you need the scale to give you permission to feel good about yourself? The way your clothes fit, what you see in the mirror, and the movement of your body are all you need to appreciate the changes in your body. Even if the number on the scale does make you feel good, the feeling is usually only temporary, and that good feeling may lead you to reward yourself throughout the day with sweet treats. Then you may get on the scale the next morning and find that it's up four pounds— not so sweet.

Now let's talk about your daughter and the scale. If you have a scale in your home, your daughter is or will be getting on it. Most young girls are. Researchers at Iowa State University found that 60 percent of the ten-year-olds were weighing themselves daily.[9] Some young women weigh themselves, others are weighed by their mothers.

"My mother puts me on the scale every morning and has a journal of my weight that goes back five years." Marsha is only twelve years old. Her mother has been weighing her since her seventh birthday, and Marsha will do just about anything to prevent negative comments from her mother. She dehydrates herself, makes sure she has a bowel movement before getting on the scale, doesn't eat breakfast until after her weigh-in, tampers with the scale so that it's off by a few pounds, and has discovered that if she shifts her weight a little to the left, the needle on the scale shifts with her and she weighs one and a half pounds less. It takes some women years to figure out these scale tricks, but Marsha and other young women are learning quickly.

When you stop weighing yourself and your daughter, you still have another scale to be aware of—the doctor's scale. Being weighed at the doctor's office can be a traumatic experience. Not only do you always seem to weigh more on the doctor's scale than on your bathroom scale, you are also reprimanded (sometimes, ironically, by an overweight doctor) for any excess poundage. This leads many of us to fast the day before an annual exam so we will weigh a bit less or, even worse, delay our appointments until we weigh a lot less. With this mentality, some annual appointments may be delayed for years.

Now, height and weight measurements are important in infancy and early childhood because they allow a physician to assess such conditions as failure to thrive and growth hormone problems. But if your daughter is six or seven and starting to comment negatively about her body, call her doctor before her appointment. Explain to her or him your concerns and ask that your daughter not be weighed. If the doctor insists on weighing her, find a new doctor.

The same strategy holds true for you at the doctor's office. Decline the weigh-in—it's your right. Tell your doctor the last measurement of your percent body fat (if you are lucky, she or he may have incorporated body fat testing into the exam), your clothing size, or give him or her your own assessment of your weight, saying that your weight is slightly up, significantly down, or about the same. When the scale is no longer important to you, you probably won't even care whether the doctor weighs you or not.

If you and/or your daughter are scale dependent, try these strategies for scaling down the importance of the scale:

1. Taper your weigh-ins by getting on once a day, then once every other day, then once a week, and so on.

2. Go cold turkey if that fits your personality better.

3. Weigh yourself many times during the day and plot your weight as suggested earlier in this section.

4. Develop a more intellectual relationship with the scale by being knowledgeable of the many factors that affect weight and how weight fluctuates throughout the day.

5. Give the scale to a charitable organization, sell it at a garage sale, or bury it in your backyard. As long as you and your scale are under the same roof, it will beckon you.

6. Beat on the scale instead of beating on yourself. One of my clients literally did beat on the scale. She put on protective goggles, took out the hammer, and went at it for fifteen therapeutic minutes. As she said, "It was the most freeing experience of my life!!"

7. Instead of getting on the scale, look at your body (preferably naked) in the mirror and ask yourself how you are feeling today. Is your body the same, larger, or smaller? Do you feel fit, muscular, and/or lean? Or do you feel sluggish, overweight, and/or bloated? If you are in touch with your body, you don't need the scale to confirm whether you've lost or gained weight.

8. If you do need some type of external measurement of your body, I recommend using measurements of your bust, waist, hips, and thighs or having your percentage of body fat analyzed. But beware of body fat testing—it can become a substitute for the scale. I once had a client who wanted her percent body fat checked every week. First of all, you can't measure body fat changes in a week; and more important, striving to reach a certain unrealistic percentage of body fat is just as self-destructive as striving to reach an unrealistic weight.

If you've already given up the scale, congratulations! It's not easily achieved, but it is an important step in changing your relationship with your body. Without the scale, you and your daughter no longer have that morning reminder that you aren't thin enough, good enough, or disciplined enough—and together, you can learn to appreciate and respect the bodies you were born with.

WORK AS A TEAM TO BUILD BODY IMAGE AND SELF-ESTEEM

Last night, I sat my daughter down for a long female body talk. We talked about how we feel about our bodies and what we can do to accept and appreciate them. I think I learned just as much from her as she did from me.

—Kim, age 41

In addition to dispelling the ideal body image set by society, finding comfort in your healthy weight, and giving up the scale, I have some further advice to help you and your daughter work as a team to build more positive body images and stronger self-esteems. The more proactive we become in promoting body acceptance, the less likely it is that we and our daughters will be lured into the trap of dieting. The Melpomene Institute and *Shape* magazine conducted a joint study on 3,800 young women ages eleven to seventeen and found that those with positive body images were *seventeen times* less likely to think they needed to diet.[10]

To break free from dieting and recapture body acceptance, focus on the following body image strategies:

MINIMIZE BEAUTY MESSAGES

Teach your daughter to value all facets of herself, not just looks or weight. Compliment her on her ideas, skills, talents, abilities, eagerness to learn, spontaneous nature, playfulness, and sense of humor.

I realize that it is tempting to tell your daughter how physically beautiful she is, but if beauty messages are not balanced with recognition of other attributes, she will come to value her looks more than her intellect, creativity, physical strength, character, and personality.

Downplay beauty messages, emphasize the development of her deeper qualities by complimenting her inner strengths, and, better yet . . .

ENCOURAGE YOUR DAUGHTER
TO COMPLIMENT HERSELF

Teach her to be her own source of positive reinforcement and self-esteem by helping her create a list of what she feels are her qualities, strengths, and skills, then periodically have her add to this self-appreciation list.

On a personal note, as someone who once relied primarily on external validation for self-worth, I now realize that the most important and lasting validation is what I think of myself, not what others think of me. I was so busy making sure that my parents thought I was smart, my teachers thought I was gifted, my friends thought I was kind, my male companions thought I was attractive, and my seminar attendees thought I was a good speaker—that I didn't have any time to make sure that I felt good about myself or believed I had any of these attributes.

RESPECT YOUR BODY

I firmly believe that we must first respect our bodies before we will treat them well with food, movement, and all else that makes us feel good. Trying to change your body is not respecting it. Respect and take care of your body first, and the change will follow—or—maybe you'll decide that you don't want to change it at all. *Improving your body image isn't about changing your body, it's about accepting it and taking care of it.*

What makes you feel good? What makes you feel bad? Do you take care of yourself when you feel tired or ill? Do you fulfill your basic needs daily?

I've had a number of clients who have realized that it has been years since they have taken care of their basic needs. They delay going to the bathroom, they don't get enough sleep at night, and they don't drink the fluids or eat the food they need to function well. If they can't take the time to restore themselves with rest and fuel, how are they going to find the time to treat themselves well with exercising, hot baths, or other nurturing care?

Teach your daughter to take care of herself by taking care of yourself. If you take care of your own physical needs, she'll get the message that her body is worthy of care. If you don't, she'll get the opposite message—that her body is not worth the time or effort.

APPRECIATE YOUR BODY

As you begin to respect and take care of yourself, an appreciation of what your body does for you every day will come naturally. But while you're still learning this behavior, do an activity with your daughter that will help you both to appreciate your bodies in a way that focuses more on function than beauty. Together, write down ten statements of body appreciation. For example, "I appreciate my strong thighs" or "I appreciate my body's flexibility." No buts allowed—meaning no negatives attached at the end of your positive statements such as "I appreciate my strong thighs, but there's too much cellulite on top of my developed muscles."

If you find that it is difficult for you to "think in positives" because throughout the years your brain has been conditioned to function only in negatives, try putting any self-deprecating comments into perspective. For example:

Self-Deprecating/ Negative	Body Appreciating/ Positive
I hate my thighs.	Larger thighs run in my family.
I despise these love handles.	I carry more weight in my hips, as all women do.
My stomach is flabby.	My stomach has extra fat and loose skin because of two pregnancies.

CELEBRATE WOMANHOOD

You have hundreds of reasons to celebrate being a woman (many of which have been shared in this and the previous chapter), and there are hundreds of ways to do so. Spend a day with your daughter just to walk and talk together about what's going on in your own and other women's lives, get together with female friends on a regular basis, form a women's book group, join a women's discussion group, go to a women's health conference, buy books written for and by women, or participate in community activities that support women.

Simply being a woman is a call for celebration! After all, for the first six weeks, all embryos are female—then only the lucky ones get to keep their female status!

WORK TOGETHER, BUT PUT *YOUR* BODY FIRST

Not only to set an example, but to enable you to be more effective in helping your daughter. It's like the airline safety instructions before the plane takes off. In case of a loss of cabin pressure, you are instructed to put your air flow mask in place first, then your children's. This advice is necessary because a mother's instinct in an emergency is to risk her life to save her children's. You may consider disordered eating and poor body image an emergency (and it is) and immediately try to give first aid to your daughter—but your efforts will mend your daughter's injured body image only temporarily because you have to have *a healthy relationship with your own body first.*

I purposely use the phrase "healthy relationship with your own body" because we need to distinguish between a "healthy body" and a "healthy relationship with our body." By society's definition, having a healthy body means one free of disease and illness—and also practically free of fat. But having a healthy relationship with our body means respecting, appreciating, and celebrating it, and, just like any other relationship in our life, fostering nurturance and acceptance of both its strengths and weaknesses.

Once you start thinking in terms of achieving a healthy relationship with your *body,* the next step of achieving a healthy relationship with *food* should come easily. Your mother-daughter body revolution has put society's thin ideal, the media pressure, and the tyranny of scale in perspective; now it's time for a revolutionary change in the way you view food, calories, and the definition of healthy eating. It's time for your declaration of food independence!

CHAPTER SIX

EMANCIPATION FROM EMACIATION: THE DECLARATION OF FOOD INDEPENDENCE

I *magine all of* the mothers and daughters of the world coming together for a buffet dinner experiment. With hidden cameras at the buffet line and dining tables, three distinct groups of women would be identified based on their eating behaviors and food choices.

The breakdown would go something like this: about 40 percent of the mothers and daughters would tentatively go through the buffet line, mentally calculating the calorie and fat content of every entree, salad, and dessert. They would choose only the "nutritionally correct" low-fat and low-calorie dishes, load up their plates with salads, and opt for the fruit plate for dessert. Although they might be tempted by various delectable entrees, they would find the will-power to resist them. At the end of the meal, most of these women would feel deprived and unsatisfied—and some would stop at McDonald's or the equivalent on the way home.

An equal percentage of women would go through the buffet

line eagerly, disregarding nutritional quality and instead going for quantity as they try to get more than their money's worth. This second group might be just as calorie conscious and weight conscious as the first group, but they would use the special social event to rationalize huge portions, seconds, and a variety of desserts. At the end of the meal, most of the women in this group would feel stuffed and guilty, and some would vow to start a new diet on their way home.

The remaining 20 percent of the mothers and daughters would go confidently through the buffet line without a thought to either cost or calories. They would take only those dishes that would be most satisfying to them and pass on all others. At the end of the meal, all of these women would feel perfectly comfortable, satisfied, and guilt-free. Some would even have food left on their plates. On their way home, these women would talk about what a good time they had.

This may be an imaginary scenario, but the results of a combination of studies have shown that on any given day approximately:

- 40% of all women are restrained eaters who restrict their food intake and deny themselves food pleasure
- 40% are overeaters who overindulge in their food desires (when they are not dieting) and feel guilty after eating, and
- 20% are instinctive eaters who eat a moderate amount of exactly what they want without a trace of guilt

Which category best describes your eating behavior? Which describes your daughter's? Which describes your mother's?

Most mothers and daughters fall into the same eating categories, while a few are in opposite categories. We either follow directly in our mother's footsteps or carve a completely different path as we rebel and search for individuality. Of course, restraint and overeating are seldom static—we vacillate back and forth because restraint causes overindulgence, and overindulgence causes restraint. We may restrain our eating today, overindulge tomorrow, and restrain again the next day. Whether we are restrained eaters, overeaters, or both, dozens of national surveys have found that women and young girls have an unrealistic definition of healthy eating, are denying themselves food pleasure, and are feeling guilty when they do eat.

Adult Women	Young Girls
50% feel guilty after eating.[1]	50% feel guilty after eating.[2]
60% believe that every food choice should be low in fat.[3]	81% believe that they have to avoid fat to have a healthy diet.[4]
More than 50% say that their eating experience is devoid of pleasure.[5]	71% believe that their favorite foods are not good for them.[6]

The truth is: We can eat some fat, we can indulge in our favorite foods, and we don't have to feel guilty about it! We can become middle-of-the-road instinctive eaters who neither restrain nor overeat! And this will be the healthy eating legacy we pass on to our daughters. But in order for this to happen, we need first to change our attitudes so that we view food as a neutral ally and eating as a morally neutral activity.

FOOD ATTITUDE ADJUSTMENT

I told my mother that I was stuffed and she went into a ten-minute sermon on the perils of overeating. I finally had to stop her and tell her that I was "stuffed" because I had a cold, not because I ate too much.

—Christina, age 15

Your attitudes about food and eating are apparent to your daughter in the kitchen, dining room, grocery store, restaurant—anytime and anywhere there is a reference to food. They are affecting the way you nourish your daughter and the way your daughter nourishes herself. If you think that overeating is a sin, fat is an evil, and willpower is a virtue, then your daughter is growing up with these same attitudes imprinted in her mind.

To get the most out of this chapter, you need to become aware of both your own food attitudes and behaviors and those of your daughter. The following self-evaluation quiz will help you to increase your awareness. Answer "yes" or "no" to the following ten questions, then have your daughter do the same.

DO YOU NEED SOME LATITUDE IN YOUR FOOD ATTITUDE?

	YOU	YOUR DAUGHTER
1. Does your weight determine how much you'll eat that day?	_____	_____
2. Do you restrict calories?	_____	_____
3. Do you restrict grams of fat?	_____	_____
4. Do you think your favorite foods are bad for you?	_____	_____
5. Do you deny yourself food when you are hungry?	_____	_____
6. Do you often skip meals?	_____	_____
7. Do you label foods as "good" or "bad"?	_____	_____
8. Do you feel uncomfortable eating in front of others?	_____	_____
9. Do you often feel out of control with your eating?	_____	_____
10. Do you often feel guilty after eating?	_____	_____
TOTAL # OF "YES" ANSWERS	_____	_____

If you and/or your daughter answered seven to ten of these questions "yes," then a combined effort to change your food attitudes is vital. If your score was three to six, then you may have already begun changing your attitudes and behaviors around food. If your score was less than three, then you have a healthy relationship with food and consider eating a morally neutral activity. You are also likely to be at a comfortable, healthy weight.

After one mother-daughter pair completed this questionnaire (each scoring nine), the mother was baffled. "I don't understand. We've been trying so hard to have a healthy diet. We've been avoiding fat, sugar, salt, and red meat—and including more fruits, vegetables, and fiber. I guess we just don't have enough willpower, discipline, and self-control."

Unfortunately, these three words—*willpower, discipline,* and *self-control*—have become our guiding principles of healthy eating. They surface in every initial counseling session I have with women who think their lack of these characteristics is responsible for their food and weight struggles. But, in reality, the opposite is true. These characteristics trigger unhealthy eating behaviors because they all cause the same struggle: trying to resist temptation and feeling inadequate when we fail. When we strive for willpower, we evaluate ourselves as "good" when we have it and "bad" when we don't. We either have the willpower to walk by the box of chocolates in our office that day or we don't and proceed to eat the entire pound; we're either in control of our food choices or food is in control of us.

Our futile search for willpower has caused 80 percent of us to vacillate between restrained eating and overeating. We're supposed to have the willpower to restrict, deprive, eliminate, omit, cut down, avoid, and reduce fat, sugar, and salt. But we can't seem to find it. And just the sound of those ominous words is enough to drive anyone to eat. It may drive you to eat a lot—in secret. With the growth of a kind of eating morality and food fundamentalism in our society, we don't seem to be admitting our difficulties with restrictive eating rules and are being less than honest with our food intake. Over the last few years, what we say we are eating and what we are really eating doesn't match up.[7]

What We Say We're Eating	What We're Really Eating
60% of us say that we are eating fewer sweets.	We are eating 9 pounds more sugar per person per year.

114

75% of us say that we are eating more fruit.	Fruit consumption has decreased 4 pounds per person per year.
70% of us say we are eating less fast food.	The number of fast food customers has increased 6%.
55% of us say that we are eating less butter.	Consumption has stayed steady.
56% of us say we are eating less ice cream.	Consumption has stayed steady.
44% of us say that we are eating more seafood.	Consumption has stayed steady.

When you remove the words "willpower," "discipline," and "self-control" from your food vocabulary, stop trying to apply the single principle of resisting temptation meant by each, and replace them with the realistic guiding principles of *variety, moderation,* and *balance,* your eating habits will become healthier. You'll no longer be bingeing on forbidden foods (secretively or otherwise), and, more important, you'll have a healthier relationship with food. There is a difference between achieving a "healthy diet" and fostering a "healthy relationship with food."

Think of someone you know who has the perfect, healthy diet. What does she eat? Colette thought of a friend. "She is a strict vegetarian, never eats processed foods, fat, or sugar, and shops only in health food stores." When I asked Colette if that was the way she wanted to eat, she replied, "No! I wouldn't last two days on a nonfat, sugar-free diet that's high in wood pulp and grass."

Now think of someone you know who has a healthy relationship with food. What does she eat? This time Colette thought of another friend. "She eats fat sometimes, and sugar sometimes, and vegetables sometimes, and red meat sometimes—I guess she eats everything—sometimes. The only thing she doesn't do sometimes is diet."

REAL WOMEN DON'T DIET

I've been dieting for so long that I diet without even thinking about it. Dieting is my security blanket; I don't know who I would be if I gave it up.

—Loretta, age 49

Many women are tentative about giving up dieting, but it's not just dieting we have to give up—it's all the thoughts and behaviors that go along with dieting. Dieting has become so pervasive in our culture that we are exhibiting the diet mentality when we're not actively dieting, and so are our daughters. The Wellesley Center for Research on Women studied the behaviors and attitudes of sixth-grade dieting and nondieting girls in Boston suburbs. I was most surprised to learn just how many nondieting girls were avoiding fat, concerned about calories, and feeling guilty after eating.[8]

	Dieting Girls (percentage)	Nondieting Girls (percentage)
Avoid fattening foods	91	46
Think too much about food	72	54
Think about calories	83	38
Eat less in front of others	85	62
Feel guilty after eating	81	27
Feel guilty after overeating	88	50

Even if your daughter is not actively dieting, she still may be avoiding foods, thinking too much about what she will and will not eat throughout the day, eating less in front of others (and more in private), and feeling guilty after she does eat. **We have to give up dieting and the dieting mentality!**

How do you become a truly nondieting female in both thought and action and help your daughter at the same time? First, realize that you will not transform yourself into a nondieter overnight. The more diets you've been on, the longer the transformation will take;

and the remaining chapters will give you continued guidance. But in the meantime, this is what you can do today:

DESIGNATE EVERY MONDAY "NATIONAL STOP DIETING DAY"

Monday is the infamous day of the week for female dieters because 99 percent of all diets are started on this back-to-work, back-to-school day. Have you ever started a diet on Friday night? It's unheard of. "Thank God It's Friday" really means "Thank God I Can Eat Again." An estimated 25,000 women start some type of diet every Monday, and 15,000 stop five days later. I wish we would stop forever, but each year provides fifty-one more Mondays to start again—unless we make dieting and Mondays mutually exclusive. While we're at it, we might as well ban dieting from our New Year's resolutions too.

PUT THE BLAME ON DIETING

We blame ourselves for our dieting failures, unhealthy body weights, and disordered eating behaviors, but the real culprit is repeated dieting. We've spent most of our lives thinking that we have eating problems when, in fact, we've had dieting problems. This is what dieting and its mentality are doing to us and our gender:

- One out of every three women is overweight.
- One out of every ten women has an eating disorder.
- Eight out of every ten women are disordered eaters—either under-eating or overeating.
- Nine out of ten women have a poor body image.

Instead of blaming ourselves and thinking that we need to try another diet, let's turn it around and start blaming dieting. When you do, you'll know that another diet is the *last* thing you need.

Self-Blame	Diet-Blame
I'm gaining weight, so I need to diet.	I'm gaining weight because I've dieted.
I'm out of control, so I need to diet.	I'm out of control because I've dieted.
I'm overeating, so I need to diet.	I'm overeating because I've dieted.

Dieting, not a lack of willpower or self-control, is the *cause* of overindulgence. In fact, just being reminded about dieting can cause us to overeat. A study at Williams College had three groups of weight-conscious women watch the movie *Terms of Endearment*. One group saw no commercials, one group saw food commercials, and the last group saw diet commercials. Would you like to guess which group ate the most during the movie? The diet commercial group not only ate more, they ate *twice* as much as the other two groups.[9]

DON'T BE SEDUCED BY DIET CLAIMS, PROMISES, AND GUARANTEES

Magazine advertisements and late-night weight-loss infomercials are so convincing that we are compelled to pick up the phone right then and there. Of course, that's the advertisers' goal. They base their claims on the assumption that impulse dieters will believe the testimonials (which are often paid for), pseudoscience jargon, and celebrity endorsements. Plus, a money-back guarantee gives us a final persuasive push to take out our credit card. We think it's worth a try especially if we can get our money back, but advertisers know that only a small percentage of dissatisfied customers will take the time to go through the complicated process of claiming reimbursement.

The most pervasive and persuasive weight-loss claims today are for diet pills and their cousins, the fat-burning pills—and, in particular, for chromium picolinate. The ads boasting that this miracle pill will build muscle and burn fat are everywhere. Chromium is necessary for muscle function, but unless you have a chromium deficiency (which is virtually nonexistent), taking this pill will not have any effect. The claim that chromium has fat-burning properties has no scientific basis at all.[10]

If you know of someone who has lost weight with chromium picolinate, find out the real story, as I did with my sixteen-year-old client. "My mom, my sister, and I are all taking this chromium fat-burning pill to lose weight, but it's only working for me." As it turned out, she was the only one exercising, and it was the exercise that was responsible for her weight loss, not the chromium picolinate.

The Food and Drug Administration has recently announced its approval of a new anti-obesity drug, Redux (or dexfenfluramine), that is believed to increase the feeling of fullness and satisfaction by altering levels of brain chemicals. Because it's too early to draw any firm conclusions, most health professionals suggest caution until long-term studies confirm the drug's efficacy and safety.

The same holds true for a potential diet pill of the future, Orlistat, a fat-blocking pill that prevents fat from being digested and absorbed. The hope is that we can eat those french fries and onion rings and corn fritters—and still lose weight. It sounds too good to be true because maybe it is. If the fat is not digested and absorbed, where does it go?

One of the participants in a clinical trial at Cornell University answered this question best: ". . . sometimes when you take the pill, you've got to be near a bathroom!"[11] The fat goes directly and quickly into the toilet, and takes any fat-soluble vitamins you've eaten along with it.

Some of my clients confuse Orlistat with the new fat substitute, Olestra, recently approved by the Food and Drug Administration. Orlistat is a pill (not yet FDA approved); Olestra is a manufactured oil that will be added to certain foods and/or used for deep-frying. Both work similarly by reducing the absorption of fat (Olestra's molecular shape is too large to be absorbed). And, therefore, both can cause diarrhea and gastrointestinal distress. They are also not likely to be the breakthrough solution to weight loss. Artificial sweeteners haven't aided our weight-loss efforts, so why should fake fats? Past varieties of diet pills haven't resulted in permanent weight loss, so why should future ones?

It seems as if a new diet pill hits the market almost every

month. It may be an herb, nutrient, hormone, or antidepressant (some are being advocated for appetite control), but a magical pill or potion for weight loss has never existed and probably never will. When we watch movies of the wild, wild West, we laugh at the snake-oil salesmen, wondering how anyone could be so gullible to believe that snake oil cured all ills. When movies are made of the booming 1980s and stressful '90s, our future relatives will be laughing at us too, wondering how we could be so gullible to believe the claims of diet pills and fad diets.

LAUGH AWAY THE DIET MENTALITY

Laughter has always been the best medicine. Here are some of Cathy Guisewite's "Cathy" comics and other clever jokes that have helped me to laugh away the diet mentality. I hope that they provide the same comic relief for your family.

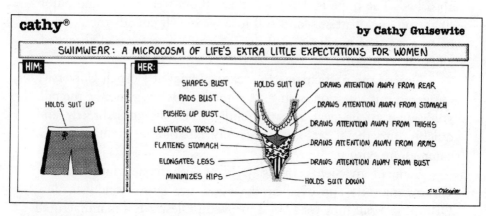

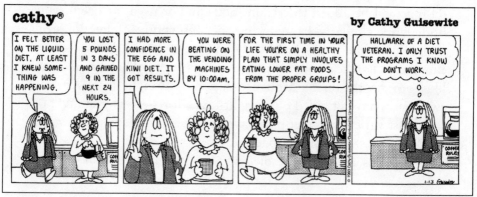

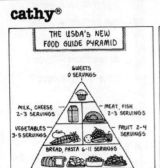
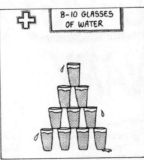
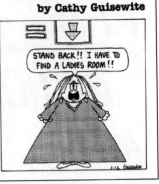
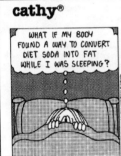
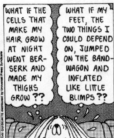
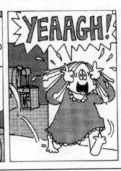
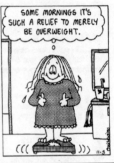
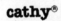
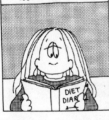
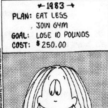
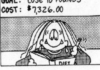
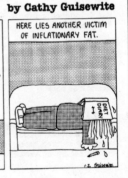
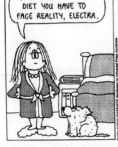
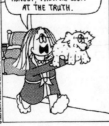
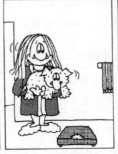
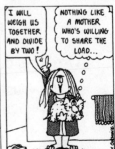

I-HATE-TO-DIET DICTIONARY

Trying to lose weight can be heavy...why not lighten the self-deprivation with this spirit-lifting lexicon?

By Sandra Bergeson

A Aerobics. *n.* A wiggling, jiggling, giggling class of moaning, groaning, toning klutzes

B Baby fat, *n.* Appealingly pudgy condition of infants, children, and young adults (not applicable after age nineteen)

C Celery, *n.* Effective low-calorie device for scraping out the last morsel of peanut butter

D Dieter, *n.* Someone never caught in the act of eating

E Exhibitionist. *n.* A size 7 who tries on clothes in a community dressing room

F Fit. *n.* Emotional outburst when jeans won't zip

G Goal. *n.* To be ten pounds less than one's ideal weight so one can have the joy of gaining it all back

H Hip, *n.* One of two protruding parts of the body used to carry small children, grocery bags, or large cartons of Twinkies

I Interested. *adj.* Telling someone else how much weight you have lost on your diet

J Justice, poetic, *n.* Attending one's tenth reunion and discovering that the ninety-pound cheerleader ... the one with the most to gain ... did

L Lockjaw. *n.* Serious illness most dieters would like to have two to three days per week

M Marquis de Sade, *n.* Eighteenth-century inventor of Nautilus equipment

N New Year's Eve. *n.* Rollicking conclusion of the old year, when one makes a sincere resolution to lose fifteen pounds by January 23

O Optimist. *n.* Any dieter who buys a leotard with horizontal stripes

P Pound. *n.* 1: a fixed unit of measure found on one's scale (usually accurate) 2: a fictitious unit of measure found on one's driver's license (usually inaccurate)

Q Quest, *n.* Everlasting pursuit of the perfect pizza

R Refrigerator, *n.* Temporary storage area between grocery bags and the mouth

S Scissors. *n.* Handy tool used to cut one-self out of photographs

T Thyroid. *n.* 1: Overactive: God's gift to Adam 2: Underactive: God's gift to Eve

U Unconscious. *adj.* The only state in which a dieter is not hungry

W Weight. *n.* Physical defiance of Newton's Law of Gravity; what goes up does not necessarily come down

Y Yin & Yang, *n.* Buddhist terms of opposition taken from the Zen macrobiotic diet 1: Yin: the loss of forty-five pounds 2: Yang: the loss of one pound, forty-five times

Z Zzzzzzz. *n.* The sound of a dieter not eating

In addition to laughing at the insight of cartoonists and authors, laughing at ourselves can also be good diet therapy. Share with your daughter the most ridiculous diet you've ever been on as well as some of the zaniest diets my clients have been on, including:

- **The Pig-Out Diet**—only pork products allowed

- **The Juggler's Diet**—you had to juggle the food to burn calories before you ate it

- **The Baby Food Diet**—jars of baby food were supposed to bring out your inner child to help you lose weight
- **The Chili Pepper Diet**—hot chili peppers had to be sprinkled over everything to increase your body temperature and boost metabolism
- **The Nutrisex Diet**—you had to make love after every meal to burn the calories before they were stored. (Sounds like one of the more satisfying diets, but you may or may not want to share this one with your daughter.)

As you are giving up dieting, a good sense of humor may be your best strategy for keeping dieting thoughts at bay.

DIVORCE DIETING AND FIND A NEW RELATIONSHIP WITH FOOD

If having a healthy relationship with food is the goal, then a divorce from dieting is warranted. We can cite irreconcilable differences and part ways. If you can't divorce yourself from dieting today, then at least do a trial separation. For the next month, decide that you, dieting, and the diet mentality are going to live in separate dwellings. See what it feels like and explore what happens. My guess is that you will want to keep away from dieting because you will have found a new, more satisfying relationship with food, one that is not focused on deprivation, restriction, counting grams of fat, or counting calories.

IN SEARCH OF THE CALORIC TRUTH

I've reduced my fat calories to almost nothing and now I'm cutting carbohydrate calories. How low should I go?
—*Laurie, age 27*

What is the real story on calories? Are fat calories the most fattening? Or are carbohydrate calories the culprit in weight gain? Are too many calories responsible for the obesity problem, or too few? Do they count or don't they? And should we be counting them?

The real story is: Calories do count because both undereating and overeating cause weight gain—but don't bother counting them. You'll only be wasting valuable time and energy that you could be using on the treadmill, with your kids, at the movies, or in the bathtub soaking away the day's stresses.

No one can tell you or your daughter how many calories a day you need to be eating to maintain, lose, or gain weight because nobody knows for sure. We all need a different number of calories and that number changes each and every day. On some days you may need 2,500 calories, on others you may need 1,500. On some days your daughter may need 5,000 calories if she is in a growth spurt, on others she may need only 1,000.

Despite this caloric variability, frustrated women have demanded, "I have to know the exact number of calories I need a day. There must be a way to find out." There is a machine called a calorimeter, if you can find it and if you have the money and time. It measures the amount of heat your body produces as it's metabolizing calories. And that's all a calorie is—a measure of heat. But you have to be locked inside the calorimeter for a week with no human contact, movement, or exposure to sunlight.

I can't tell you how many calories you need to eat to lose weight, but what I can tell you is that many of us are eating too few calories. Based on the latest nutrition assessments, the average adult woman consumes only 1,468 calories a day—or about what a twenty-nine-pound toddler needs daily[12]—and doesn't lose weight. In another study, more than 50 percent of the college-age females reported eating fewer than 600 calories at least one day during the previous month[13]—and wondered why the pounds weren't melting away.

You don't have to wonder any longer. The accepted energy balance equation seldom works as expected. This equation states that if your calorie input is less than your calorie output, you'll lose weight. If it worked predictably, we would all have lost weight years ago. It may work in a test tube, but not in our bodies.

3,500 CALORIES DOES *NOT* EQUAL ONE POUND

I'm sure you've heard and been motivated by a statement like this: "If you cut 300 calories a day, you'll lose thirty pounds in a year." The promise is based on the premise that it takes 3,500 calories to gain or lose a pound. It sounds convincing enough—but any motivation will be short-lived because cutting calories may cause weight gain instead of weight loss as metabolism drops and your brain fights against your efforts.

Your brain is your body's expert calorie accountant. It figures out how many calories all of your organs need that day to keep you alive and well and assesses whether you are in the black or the red. If you're in the red, it does what it needs to do to make sure that your organs are functioning—and you don't lose weight.

For example, if you are dieting and eat a salad with nonfat dressing for lunch, your brain will go through a series of accounting steps. "All right. I guess she's done eating this measly salad. Let's see, that's 267 calories. Here's 108 calories for the heart, 56 calories for the kidneys, 87 calories for the lungs. . . . Damn! She's done it again and hasn't eaten enough. I have nothing left for her other organs. Well, my only alternative is to conserve calories by slowing down the metabolism of every cell and organ so that she can stay alive on 267 calories until she eats again."

FAT-FREE IS *NOT* CALORIE-FREE

Have you experienced the enigma of nonfat weight gain? You are buying everything from nonfat salad dressings to nonfat chocolate cookies—and your weight is defying the law of nutrition and curiously creeping up the scale.

If you are overeating nonfat foods (most people are), then weight gain is inevitable and understandable because you're consuming more calories than your body needs. With an overemphasis on the fat content of the diet, there has been an underemphasis on total calorie intake. We have been led to believe that we can eat as much as we want as long as it doesn't contain fat. Gram for gram, fat does contain over twice as many calories as carbohydrates and protein: fats contain 9 calories per gram, while carbohydrates and protein contain 4 calories per gram. But the problem is that most fat-free foods have just as many calories as the regular versions because carbohydrates are added in place of the fat.

Next time you are in the grocery store, do some comparison shopping. Look at the food labels of the regular version and nonfat version and compare calories and carbohydrates. Many of the nonfat foods are similar in calorie content; some are even higher. Here are a few examples:

- Fat-Free Fig Newtons contain 110 calories per serving; so do the regular Fig Newtons.
- Jell-O Fat-Free Instant Chocolate Pudding and regular Jell-O Instant Pudding have 140 calories per serving.
- Reduced Fat Jif Peanut Butter and the regular Jif both have 190 calories per serving. They removed 4 grams of fat and added 7 grams of carbohydrate as well as 100 extra milligrams of sodium.
- Betty Crocker Supermoist Light Devils Food Cake Mix contains 210 calories per serving, but the regular version has only 190 calories per serving.

Even if a nonfat food is significantly lower in calories, the calories can quickly add up to extra pounds. Entenmann's Fat-Free Fudge Brownie Cake may have only 110 calories per serving, but that's only for 1/10th of the cake. Why stop at a small sliver when it's fat-free? If we eat the whole thing, 1,100 fat-free calories will be converted to fat and stored as fat. And some of us *are* eating the whole thing. One client told me that she was now eating nonfat chocolate cake and was quite proud of her dietary change. When I asked how much nonfat cake she was eating, she replied, "Oh, usually one or two." I thought she was referring to one or two pieces until she finally clarified, "Oh, no, I'm not eating one or two pieces; I'm eating one or two cakes."

Don't let fat-free translate into guilt-free permission to eat. Instead, focus on the overall amount of food that you are eating and how you feel after eating. If you feel uncomfortably full after eating industrial-size portions of fat-free foods, your body is converting the carbohydrates and protein in those foods to fat and storing them as fat. As long as they are satisfying and you don't overeat them, fat-free foods are fine—but if you are overeating them, a calorie is a calorie is a calorie.

PASTA DOES *NOT* MAKE YOU FAT

After all the hard work nutritionists have done to reclaim the good reputation that starches deserve, one recent *New York Times* headline that read "So It May Be True After All: Eating Pasta Makes You Fat" brought us back to the dieting dark ages.[14] And since then, hundreds of women have asked me: Does pasta go straight to the hips? Is bread really fattening? Are potatoes the worst thing a couch potato can eat? Should I restrict my and my daughter's starch intake?

The answer is "no"; it's not true after all, and we shouldn't restrict starches. If pasta and other starches made us fat, I would be overweight right now, and so would all other fit people who focus on carbohydrates. The government would be revising its recommendation of having six to eleven servings of grains a day in the new Food Guide Pyramid.

The "science" behind the *New York Times* story and a number of weight-loss books is that carbohydrates increase insulin levels, and this hormone causes fat storage. Those people who are insulin resistant produce more insulin in response to carbohydrates and, therefore, are more likely to store fat and put on a few pounds with pasta.

But this reaction is *only* true if you overeat pasta or any other high-starch food. Overweight people are more likely to be resistant to insulin, but most scientists agree that the insulin resistance didn't cause the weight gain—the weight gain caused the insulin resistance.[15] How can reputable newspapers and magazines report less than the whole picture? They can—and they do.

NUTRITION ADVICE THAT'S HARD TO SWALLOW

> *My mother read in a magazine that when you eat in the kitchen with other people, you automatically eat more calories. So she imprisoned us in our bedrooms during meals as a weight-loss strategy.*
>
> *—Sandy, age 21*

How does the saying go? "Believe a quarter of what you hear, a third of what you read, and half of what you see." This saying is definitely true when it comes to nutrition advice.

Hundreds of books are written on healthy eating and hundreds of articles appear in magazines and newspapers each year. Despite the abundance of nutrition information, we're still asking the same questions: Is sugar okay or not? Is red meat still bad? Is margarine still good? Is coffee liquid death or not? Help! What's the best way to nourish myself and my family?

Even those with PhDs in nutrition are having a difficult time answering these questions because nutrition is not an exact science. It is virtually impossible to control for all factors that affect the human body and to determine a direct cause-and-effect relationship. But with cover lines stating "Breakthrough Research Shows . . ." or "New Study Finds . . ." we believe that the findings of one study are enough proof to either avoid a food for the rest of our lives or to eat it every day.

The next time you read a newspaper or magazine article reporting on the latest breakthrough study, beware of three things:

1. **Beware of animals**—look for rats, pigs, monkeys, dogs, or other laboratory animals being used as the subjects of the study. Just because a certain response has been discovered in an animal doesn't mean that it will hold true for humans.

2. **Beware of males**—even if the study used human beings as the subjects, most likely the researchers "forgot" to include women in it. Just because a specific reaction has been found to occur in males doesn't mean that the same will hold true for females.

3. **Beware of the first few paragraphs**—this is where the confusing statistics and exaggerated statements usually appear. Skip down to the last few paragraphs where outside experts usually put the study in perspective.

Where science and journalism meet is often shaky ground. A *New York Times* article recently highlighted the journalistic problems in reporting nutrition studies, and the journalist wrote, "Is it any wonder that amid all this information, Americans have let their eating habits take a turn for the worse?"[16]

No, it isn't any wonder. We don't know what to believe any longer, so we throw up our hands in defeat. Before you do that, let me dispel some accepted nutritional dogma and share some advice that's *much easier to swallow.*

1. **Eggs are *not* necessarily unhealthy.** I agree with the posters saying "Give Eggs a Break" as they are being let out of jail (unless they are uncooked or undercooked, because of the possible presence of salmonella). Eggs contain about a third less cholesterol than was previously thought, but the news gets even better. Two-thirds of us may not be sensitive to the cholesterol in foods, meaning if we eat eggs or another food high in cholesterol, our blood cholesterol levels do not significantly rise.[17] Even if we are sensitive to cholesterol, eating eggs isn't the major problem. It's the butter we scramble them in and the bacon or sausage we eat with them. Animal fat helps to transport the cholesterol into our bloodstream, so an egg scrambled in a nonstick pan and served with dry toast lacks the animal fat that's necessary to increase blood cholesterol levels.

2. **Chicken and turkey are *not* necessarily better than beef or pork.** Because the fat content of beef and pork has come down over the last few years, pork tenderloin is now just as low in fat as skinless chicken breast, and London broil is lower in fat than a chicken thigh (and a much better source of iron).

3. **Margarine is *not* necessarily better than butter.** Both margarine and butter are 100 percent fat, which makes them equals, but the newest news is definitely pro-butter: margarine is artificially

hydrogenated (which brings it from a liquid to a solid form) and may increase blood cholesterol levels just as much as butter. But with either one, use as small an amount as you can.

4. **Salt and high-salt foods do *not* necessarily increase blood pressure.** Only one-fifth of the population appears sensitive to salt; the rest of us do not experience a rise in blood pressure after we eat a high-salt food. But as too much salt is a strain on the kidneys, it's best not to go overboard.

5. **Fresh vegetables are *not* necessarily better than frozen.** Actually, the opposite may be true from a nutrient standpoint. Frozen vegetables are sealed and protected shortly after being picked and, therefore, maintain their vitamin and mineral content. Fresh vegetables in the grocery store can lose as much as 20 percent of their nutrients from exposure to the air and light.[18] If you go to a farmer's market to get your produce, the nutrient content may be higher—but then it depends on how long you keep the vegetables in the refrigerator or on the counter before you eat them.

6. **Sugar does *not* necessarily cause hyperactivity.** The FDA's Sugar Task Force reviewed all the research and found no conclusive evidence that sugar caused negative behavior changes in children or adults. If kids seem to get excited when they eat sugar, it's most likely because they are excited to finally be given permission to eat sugar. After this explanation, the mothers usually rely on the sugar/cavity connection to rationalize their anti-sugar stance. They are surprised when I tell them that raisins, bread, and other foods that stick to the teeth are just as cavity producing as sugar.[19] What's most important is brushing our teeth after we eat any carbohydrate.

7. **Fat is *not* all bad.** We all need some fat to make estrogen, to help our nervous system function, and to absorb the fat-soluble vitamins. If you have a young daughter, she needs even more fat because her brain (which is made up of 100 percent fat) is still developing. Fat is also not the culprit in weight gain it was once thought to be. One study took overweight women and assigned them to different groups where 10 percent of their calories were

coming from fat, 20 percent were from fat, 30 percent were from fat, or 40 percent were from fat. They were all taking in the same number of total calories and all exercising. No difference in weight loss or body fat loss was found among the groups.[20] Fat makes you fat only if it adds too many calories to your total diet.

So, eggs, red meat, butter, white bread, sugar, and fat are not that bad after all. Whatever foods you decide to eat and feed your family, take great care in buying, washing, and preparing them. With the recent spread in foodborne illnesses, the fresher and the higher the quality of the foods, the better.

After thirty years of nutrition research, there are only three solid areas of consensus: variety, moderation, and balance. *By eating a variety of foods in moderation and balancing our food intake, we can have the freedom to eat what we want, when we want it— and declare our individual food independence!*

THE BILL OF MOTHER–DAUGHTER FOOD RIGHTS

If I stop dieting, counting calories, and following accepted nutrition advice, how will I know what to eat and what to feed my daughter?

—*Jamie, age 38*

When you reclaim the right to:

- pleasure your taste buds with the foods you like
- fuel your body when you are hungry
- consider eating a morally neutral activity
- take the guilt out of eating and put the enjoyment back in

you'll automatically know what, when, and how much to eat—and so will your daughter. You can start reclaiming these rights with the Bill of Food Rights.

The Bill of Food Rights

1. Freedom of Food Preferences
2. Freedom of Food Choices
3. Freedom of Mealtimes
4. The Right to Bear Hips and Thighs
5. The Right to Assemble Peacefully for a Meal
6. The Right to be Free from Unreasonable Scrutiny and Suffering with Food
7. The Right to Eat What We Want in Public
8. The Right to Eat Ice Cream for Dinner
9. The Right to Dislike Broccoli
10. The Right to Not Have Perfect Eating Habits

After reading this chapter, you probably know what these rights mean, but I will explain each one briefly.

FREEDOM OF FOOD PREFERENCES

When kindergarten students were asked about their favorite foods, they listed meats, fruits, and grains among their top preferences.[21] Our and our daughters' favorite foods are not always loaded with fat and sugar, but even if they are, they are important to include in a balanced diet to satisfy our taste buds. It's perfectly normal to like french fries, to crave chocolate, or to yearn for pizza from your favorite pizza parlor.

What are your favorite foods? What are your daughters'?

Your Top 5 Favorite Foods	Your Daughter's Top 5 Favorite Foods
1._____	1._____
2._____	2._____
3._____	3._____
4._____	4._____
5._____	5._____

Acknowledge that these foods are important to you, and incorporate them into your diet. If you don't, you'll feel deprived and eat twice as much next time you get your hands on them.

FREEDOM OF FOOD CHOICES

All food choices are good choices, even those that contain fat and sugar. Food choices are supposed to change daily because our bodies' needs change daily. Some days your body may want no sugar; on other days it may want a lot of sugar. Some days you can't seem to get enough protein; on other days you could care less about protein and want vegetables. Listen to your body and choose the foods you want.

FREEDOM OF MEALTIMES

We are conditioned to eat breakfast at 7 A.M., lunch at 12 noon, and dinner at 6 P.M. If we are not hungry during these times, we eat anyway. If we are hungry during other times, we wait until the next socially accepted mealtime to give our bodies fuel. We need to start eating when our bodies tell us it's time to eat.

If clocks didn't exist, and you gave your body an opportunity to set your eating schedule, what times would you eat throughout the day? It may be 9 A.M., 1 P.M., and 5 P.M.—or it may be 6 A.M., 9 A.M., 12 P.M., 3 P.M, and 7 P.M. What times would your daughter want to eat throughout the day?

THE RIGHT TO BEAR HIPS AND THIGHS

This one doesn't have much to do with food, but I couldn't resist the wordplay. So, to emphasize the point once again, women have the biological right to be pear-shaped and to wear a larger size pants or skirt than top.

THE RIGHT TO ASSEMBLE PEACEFULLY FOR A MEAL

In 1995, the American Dietetic Association launched its Child Nutrition and Health Campaign. One of its primary goals is to put the "fun" back into food. I couldn't agree more. For adults too, I believe we need to put "fun" back into food and the "enjoyment" back into eating. When your family sits down to a meal, make it as free of anxiety, pressure, and control as possible.

THE RIGHT TO BE FREE FROM UNREASONABLE SCRUTINY AND SUFFERING FROM FOOD

We feel that the whole world is watching us eat and evaluating our food choices, but does the world really care what you are eating for dinner tonight? Certain people may give you dirty looks or make snide remarks about your food choices, but they usually need to come to terms with their own food issues. Do you act as the "diet disciplinarian" with your daughter, looking over her shoulder and criticizing her food choices? If you do, she may start to feel guilty about her food desires and become a secretive eater.

THE RIGHT TO EAT WHAT WE WANT IN PUBLIC

Our focus on calories and dieting has caused us to tell little white lies about our eating habits. It starts in childhood with such comments as "No, I didn't eat the rest of the cookies" or "I don't know how that candy wrapper got in my backpack" or "I did so finish my Brussels sprouts." As adults, we may get in the habit of secretive eating and consider drive-thrus our food haven and the car our eating sanctuary. Be honest, you're only fooling yourself. *Eat what you want in public—and you'll eat less in private.*

THE RIGHT TO EAT ICE CREAM FOR DINNER

Or anything else. We don't need to get all the four groups at dinner, and sometimes we only want ice cream for dinner. If dessert is what you or your daughter really desires for dinner, have it. You won't become malnourished overnight. Also, feel free to have breakfast foods for dinner, dinner foods for breakfast, and lunch foods for snacks—if that's what you want.

THE RIGHT TO DISLIKE BROCCOLI

Or any other food. Broccoli may be one of the more nutritious veg-etables, filled with vitamins, minerals, antioxidants, and phytochem-icals (natural disease-fighting substances), but you or your daughter may not like it. If George Bush could admit that he didn't like broc-coli, so can you. When asked about their least favorite food, 75 percent of young children named a vegetable.[22] Children prefer fruits over vegetables for a reason: their taste buds find fruit delicious and many vegetables bitter. It's more important for children to eat fruit because it provides more calories for growth.

What are your least favorite foods? What are your daughter's?

Your 5 Least Favorite Foods	**Your Daughter's 5 Least Favorite Foods**
1._____	1._____
2._____	2._____
3._____	3._____
4._____	4._____
5._____	5._____

Regardless of nutritional quality, don't force yourself or your daughter to eat foods that you or she doesn't like. Each of you will develop negative attitudes about those foods and search for satis-faction elsewhere.

THE RIGHT TO NOT HAVE PERFECT EATING HABITS

Because, I hope you'll now agree, perfect eating habits don't exist. Variety, moderation, and balance imply imperfection, giving you a range of acceptable, healthy eating behaviors.

I certainly don't have perfect eating habits. But before I went through my own declaration of food independence fifteen years ago, I tried and tried and tried. As a nutritionist, I was supposed to have a picture-perfect diet and set an example with immense amounts of willpower to stay away from my favorite foods. I shopped in health food stores and tried to condition my taste buds to live on fruits, vegetables, and whole grains. But just because I'm a nutritionist doesn't mean I'm not human. I still wanted my pizza and potato chips! I was in a nutritional dilemma. If I ate them in public, I would be labeled a "bad" nutritionist. If I didn't eat them, I knew I'd be completely dissatisfied with my diet. My solution was to eat them when no one was looking.

Today I can boldly say that I adore pizza and potato chips, and I prefer to eat them together on the same plate. I also dislike a number of foods that should disbar me from the nutrition profession, but for my nutritional sanity, I'll take my chances.

My 5 Favorite Foods	My 5 Least Favorite Foods
1. cheese pizza	1. rice
2. potato chips	2. celery
3. Swiss chard	3. okra
4. mashed potatoes with gravy	4. anything with curry
5. dark chocolate	5. chocolate with nuts

Yes, I am a nutritionist who doesn't like rice. I never have. You may find it odd (my husband finds it obsessive) that I love chocolate, but I hate chocolate with nuts in it. I describe it as heightened self-awareness of my food needs; I simply don't like the combination.

When friends witness me ordering a hamburger and french fries or when clients see my grocery cart containing potato chips, I think of it as an educational experience. They are learning that a healthy person at a comfortable weight with a generally well-balanced diet can eat some fat and sugar and not gain weight.

Each of your personal declarations of food independence will take a different course depending on your initial food attitudes and behaviors and your current food preferences and food needs. But by reclaiming your food rights, you *are* establishing a healthier relationship with food and can naturally and confidently move to the important next step of fostering a healthier food relationship with your daughter.

CHAPTER SEVEN

THE REBIRTH
OF HEALTHY
MOTHER–DAUGHTER
FOOD
RELATIONSHIPS

Y*our daughter walks* into the kitchen and confidently states, "Mom, I'm hungry. I need something to eat." When you ask her what she wants, she thinks a moment and then tells you that she wants barbecued potato chips and orange sections. While you're peeling the orange, she takes a bag of chips out of the cupboard and puts a handful on a plate. A few minutes later, she gets up from the kitchen counter, scrapes four remaining orange sections down the disposal, and heads out the door to play.

This is an example of a healthy mother-daughter food interaction—and one you can use as a model for your and your daughter's eating behavior. Regardless of her age or body weight, your daughter is the food decision maker. She decides when she needs to eat, what she needs, and how much food she needs—and you let the process take place without protest, criticisms, or comments. Up until now, when your daughter wanted a snack, you might have questioned her hunger and food choices with such comments as "No snacking before dinner" or "Potato chips are unhealthy and loaded with fat, so have some unsalted pretzels instead" or "Get back here and finish these four nutritious orange sections."

These types of food-controlling, negative comments are a thing of the past. Your new, healthy mother-daughter food relationship will be based on trust, instinct, education, and knowledge. When your daughter requests potato chips (with or without the orange sections), you have faith in her decision because she is hungry and must need the fat, starch, and salt. You also know that her food needs are constantly changing. Yesterday she might have wanted a slice of turkey breast and cheese, and tomorrow she might not want anything—because she's not hungry.

As a mother concerned about the health and welfare of your daughter, your responsibility is not to control her eating but to provide a wide variety of all types of foods and to help her make her own food decisions. If your daughter is a toddler or young child, this means putting small portions of different kinds of foods on her plate and letting her choose what and how much she eats. If she is an older child, adolescent, or teen, this means stocking a wide variety of foods in the house and permitting her to choose what and how much she eats.

Whatever her age, there are two overall goals to the rebirth of your healthy mother-daughter food relationship:

1. to trust your own eating instincts and eat in a way that's right for *your* body, and

2. to trust your daughter's eating instincts and assist her in eating in a way that's right for *her* body.

And what's right for you may be very different from what's right for your daughter. There is no right or wrong! Although each of us is unique and has special food needs, the end result is the same: You and your daughter will be free from dieting, food insecurities, and weight preoccupation. Together, you will break the chain of disordered eating by becoming instinctive eaters.

To welcome instinctive eating into your mother-daughter food relationship, you have to begin trusting and responding to your own eating messages first. Someone who doesn't know how to swim can't save a drowning person. If you don't know how to listen to your own signals for when, what, and how much you need to eat, you can't effectively teach your daughter to listen to hers.

TEACHING BY EXAMPLE: BECOMING AN INSTINCTIVE EATER

I'm trying to teach my daughter to eat what she wants when she is hungry, but yesterday she said that she wanted to be on the same diet I was on. I thought I was keeping my latest dieting attempt a secret, but she watches my every move.

—*Christine, age 43*

Some mothers think they can continue dieting, restricting, and depriving themselves while teaching their daughter to have a healthy relationship with food. But young children are perceptive. No matter how much you try to mask your behavior, your daughter will notice that you are dieting.

So, how can you begin to trust your body's messages and openly transform your relationship with food and ultimately your daughter's? Giving up all forms of dieting is the first step. After reading the first six chapters of this book, my hope is that your new motto is "Real Women Don't Diet" and that you've already given up dieting or are very close to making this important decision. Perhaps you've been waiting for the specific guidance of what to do about regulating your eating behavior when you finally stop dieting. Your waiting is over.

ASK NOT WHAT YOUR BODY CAN DO FOR YOU, ASK WHAT YOU CAN DO FOR YOUR BODY

We expect ourselves to lose weight quickly, to have energy when we haven't eaten, to have the willpower to stay away from our favorite foods, and to crave only nutritious foods. With expectations like these, we are bound to be disappointed in our bodies and ourselves.

Instead of asking your body to accomplish the impossible, start every morning asking what *you* can do to take care of your body today.

- Can you provide fuel for your body when you're hungry?
- Can you give yourself pleasure with the foods you want?
- Can you include a snack or two during the day to give yourself sustained energy?
- Can you hydrate yourself with water and other fluids?

Of course you can! And when you do, your body will give you back so much more. If you have weight to lose, you'll lose it. If you have fatigue to fight, you'll fight it. If you have a busy schedule to meet, you'll meet it. If you have mood swings to stabilize, you'll stabilize them.

As you begin paying attention to your body's needs, you'll start recognizing the signals of when, what, and how much you need to eat—and soon you'll realize how important these signals are to your physical and emotional well-being and how wonderful you feel when you respond to them and honor your hunger.

HONOR YOUR HUNGER

When you are hungry, not just your stomach but every single body cell is requesting fuel. If you deny your hunger, you are asking your cells to work on an inadequate fuel supply. But when you honor your hunger, you are supplying your brain, breasts, heart, muscles, kidneys, lungs, and all the rest of your organs with the fuel to function at optimal capacity.

Some women think of hunger as a negative feeling, and they eat to prevent it. I don't recommend that you wait until you are famished before you eat. When you are extremely hungry, you feel light-headed, irritable, and foggy—and you'll want more food and higher-calorie foods to make up for the wait. To the contrary, I recommend that you eat when the *first* hunger signals emerge.

What are your first signals of hunger? Does your stomach growl or feel empty? Do you experience a slight drop in energy? This is how you know when you are hungry, but not too hungry.

There are three parts to honoring your hunger:

1. Knowing when you are hungry

2. Knowing what you are hungry for

3. Knowing when your hunger is satisfied

Once you know that your body is signaling that it's time to eat, you need to know *what* you're hungry for. What specific food or foods will satisfy your hunger? Do you want something starchy, salty, or sugary? Do you need some protein, vegetables, calcium, or fat? Do you yearn for cheese, cranberries, carrots, caramel, or chocolate? In other words, is your body sending you a specific message through food cravings?

Food cravings—sometimes just hearing the words can bring about feelings of frustration, defeat, and failure. We have been taught that food cravings are the enemy, an unhealthy sign of weakness that must be controlled and conquered. Not any longer! Food cravings are the *only* means your body has to communicate what you need to function optimally over the next couple of hours. These messages are vital; they will tell you when you need a particular nutrient for health, when you need protein to build and repair muscle, when you need carbohydrates to give your blood sugar a boost—and when you need chocolate or another sugar/fat combination to lift your moods. (My recent book, *Why Women Need Chocolate,* explains the physiological basis of food cravings in much greater detail.)

Think about the foods that you regularly crave. Do you have specific, undeniable cravings for nonfat cheese? How about tofu? Alfalfa sprouts? Rice cakes? Most women laugh at these suggestions. We know what our bodies crave: starch, sugar, fat, chocolate, salt, and sometimes fruits, vegetables, and protein.

When your next food craving hits and you are presented with the should-I-eat-it or shouldn't-I-eat-it dilemma, give yourself guilt-free permission to fulfill your food craving. Your body is sending you this message for a specific reason. Cravings aren't the enemy, but deprivation is. If you deny the craving, it will only intensify. *Instead, let your cravings do the talking—and you'll know exactly what you're hungry for.*

So, once you know that you're hungry and know exactly what you want, the third part of honoring your hunger is knowing when your hunger is satisfied. If you don't eat enough, you haven't satisfied your hunger and your metabolism will slow down. If you eat too much, you've overeaten and satisfied your fat cells too.

Do you know the difference between satisfying your hunger and overeating? *Satisfying your hunger* means that you are no longer hungry—you've eaten the right amount to fill your stomach and take away any feelings of hunger. *Overeating* means that you have overfilled your stomach. Your waistband feels tighter, your blood supply is directed to your stomach for labored digestion, and your fat cells are anxiously awaiting that extra helping of lasagna. When you experiment with different amounts of food and give your body a chance, you'll start to recognize the difference between satisfying hunger and overeating. Perhaps until now, portion size determined the amount you were eating, not your hunger.

Trust your body to tell you when, what, and how much you need to eat to fill your stomach. One frustrated client, Diana, questioned her ability to trust. "I know I'll overeat if you don't tell me exactly how much I should be eating. I can't trust my body." Is it that you can't—or you won't? You *can* trust yourself if you choose to make it a priority and think of it as a learning process that will take time. All you need to do is start asking the right questions.

THREE QUESTIONS ARE A CHARM

The typical eating questions we ask during the course of the day are: How can I fight my hunger? What can I eat that's low in calories and fat? How can I eat as little as possible? These are the questions a dieter would ask. But an instinctive eater asks: Am I hungry? What am I hungry for? Is my hunger satisfied?

Every time you eat, ask yourself these three important questions—they are your tools for trusting your body and becoming an instinctive eater. At first, you may forget to ask the questions and remember only after you've finished eating. Some of my clients have put notes on the refrigerator or left themselves voice-mail messages to aid their short-term memory, but soon they felt so good responding to their hunger that they wanted to make sure they asked these questions. You will too! And eventually you won't have to ask them at all because your body will automatically answer them before you get a chance.

Because these three questions form the cornerstone of instinctive eating and the development of healthy mother-daughter food relationships, I will explain them in greater depth in the next section, which explains how to teach your daughter to trust her eating instincts. But as you begin to honor your hunger, ask and answer these questions out loud in your young daughter's presence. For example:

Question	Answer in Your Daughter's Presence
Am I hungry?	Did you hear my stomach growl? My stomach is telling me that it is hungry.
What am I hungry for?	Let's see, a ham sandwich would taste good to me right now.
Is my hunger satisfied?	I think I've almost had enough. One more bite ought to do it.

I will share many effective methods to teach your daughter how to trust her eating instincts, but keep in mind that your best teaching tool is *you.*

TEACHING YOUR DAUGHTER TO TRUST HER EATING INSTINCTS

*My mom isn't like other moms. She always lets me eat
what I want to, and she always makes sure that my
favorite foods are in the house.*

—*Katie, age 6*

Depending on your daughter's age, you may not have to teach her at all, but instead, you'll only need to reinforce her instinctive eating behaviors. Before young children are influenced by parents and society's eating rules, they respond instinctively to their bodies' food messages. They eat when they are hungry, play with their food when they are not, and seldom overeat.

Chances are, though, your eating behaviors and food attitudes have already influenced your daughter, and she has lost touch with her natural eating instincts. Before she can develop and maintain a healthy relationship with food, you have to let her be in charge of when, what, and how much she eats.

"What!?! You can't be serious. My daughter is out of control with her eating. If I put her in charge, she either won't eat enough or she'll eat too much." If this is your reaction to making your daughter responsible for her food decisions, your prediction probably will come true. But instead of being concerned, let me reassure you that variability is a part of instinctive eating. Because her food needs change throughout the day, sometimes your daughter will eat a lot and other times she'll eat a little.

More than sixty years ago, Clara Davis, a pioneer in child development, found over and over again that when parents refrained from controlling their children's food intake, their children perfectly adjusted their own calorie intake to their ever changing appetites and their physical development was on target. Sometimes they ate "like a bird" and other times they ate "like a horse"—but even though they ate sporadically, they consumed the exact amount of food their bodies needed.[1]

Current research has continued to support the normalcy of sporadic eating. Drs. Leana Birch and Susan Johnson at the University of Illinois have been researching children's eating behavior for many years and have consistently found that when parents allowed their children to eat the amount they wanted when they were hungry, the children adjusted their food intake to meet their caloric needs. If they ate too little at one meal or snack, they ate more at the next meal and vice versa.[2]

Children (and adults too) are supposed to be sporadic eaters with great variation in the amounts consumed at each meal or snack but little variation in the amount consumed day to day and almost none in the amount consumed week to week. *Sporadic eating is a characteristic of instinctive eating!*

To encourage this natural variability and assist your daughter in trusting her eating instincts, the same three questions are the charm:

ARE YOU HUNGRY?

Whenever she asks for food or takes food without asking, ask her this fundamental question. You may sound like a broken record, but you will be reinforcing the important message that she *can* and *should* respond to her body's hunger signals. Explain to her what hunger is, why her body needs food when she's hungry, and help her to identify her specific hunger signals.

What if you ask "Are you hungry?" and she answers, "No, not really"? Your immediate reaction may be to tell her that there is no reason to eat and she'll gain weight if she does. Although this is indeed true, don't withhold food. Forbidding her to eat is food control. She'll feel denied and will want to eat all the more later when you're not looking. Whether she is hungry or not, it's up to her to decide to eat. But you can help her make that decision by exploring why she feels the need to eat when her body doesn't need to.

- Is she really thirsty instead of hungry? Thirst signals can easily be misread as hunger signals.
- Did a commercial just come on to remind her of food?
- Is she bored watching TV?
- Does she want to eat because her friends are over and they want a snack?

- Is she having a difficult time concentrating on her homework?

- Is an emotion triggering her need to eat?

Emotional eating often starts in childhood. Parents inadvertently encourage it by giving ice cream to help stop the tears from an unhappy moment or candy to ease the pain from a skinned knee. We learn early on that certain foods comfort us—if only temporarily. The sadness and pain are still there after the food is gone.

You can reduce the likelihood of emotional eating by helping your daughter to specify *what* she is feeling. One mother said, "I have a difficult time identifying my own feelings. All I can think to ask her is if she's sad or happy." For this mother, as well as for you, the following list may help you to identify your own feelings and help your daughter identify hers. If she's not feeling hungry, ask her, "Are you feeling . . . ?"

sad	bored	lonely
frustrated	anxious	tired
embarrassed	depressed	stressed
hurt	angry	confused
guilty	ashamed	afraid

Then help her identify what she really needs. Does she need to call a friend, cry, take a nap, be active, have a drink of water? Or does she need to talk about her feelings or write them down? Give her other options besides eating, but leave the decision up to her.

When you give your daughter permission to eat when *she* decides to, some frustrating issues may come up for *you:*

- **"My daughter is never hungry in the morning and we get into heated arguments about the importance of breakfast."** Your daughter may not need food first thing in the morning, and therefore, breakfast may not be her "most important meal of the day." Trust her to trust her body and give her a snack that she can take with her to eat when she does get hungry. Or, if you are concerned that she won't get a chance to eat at school until lunchtime, wake her up a half hour earlier and give her metabolism a chance to kick into gear so that she will be hungry before she leaves.

- **"My daughter is not very hungry at dinnertime."** If she eats when she's hungry during the day, there is a good chance that she won't need a large dinner. Her body's food needs are minimal at night and a snack may be just right.

- **"My daughter says she is hungry ten times a day."** Then trust her and let her eat ten times a day. Our bodies actually prefer to eat smaller amounts more frequently throughout the day.

- **"My daughter says that she is hungry within a half hour after eating dinner."** It may be because she didn't eat quite enough to fulfill her body's food needs and realized it thirty minutes later. It may also be that she is testing you to see if you are sticking to your word that she is in charge of her food decisions. And a final explanation may be that she's in the habit of snacking at night—most of us are. The Wellesley Center for Research on Women found that 70 percent of the sixth-grade girls were snacking after dinner.[3] As your daughter becomes more of an instinctive eater, she will no longer feel the need to snack at night.

- **"My daughter says she's hungry right before bed."** She knows that those three words "Mom, I'm hungry" get your attention, and you'll stop everything to cater to her hunger. She may be using "the hunger ploy" to delay her bedtime. Ask her if she's hungry a half hour before bed, and tell her this is the time to have a snack if she needs it.

WHAT ARE YOU HUNGRY FOR?

At the beginning of this new program, your daughter will thoroughly enjoy this question, but you may find it terrifying. She will be happily pleasuring her taste buds with any food she wants while you're worrying that she'll become malnourished from eating junk food for the rest of her life. Rest assured—studies have proven that the instinctive eating approach ultimately increases her nutrient intake and decreases her consumption of sweets and fats. If you've been restricting your daughter's diet, she may overindulge for a few days. But within a week or two, she won't want to indulge in sweets or fats as often—*simply because she can have them as often as she likes.*

When Laura first started trusting her daughter's food messages, she thought her daughter, Christina, would become a jelly bean junkie. Laura used to allow jelly beans only on special occasions, and when she did, her daughter would put twenty in her mouth at once. With my recommendation, Laura bought two pounds of jelly beans, gave them to Christina, and said, "Here are jelly beans for you to eat whenever you are hungry for them. When you run out, just let me know and I'll get you some more." At first, Christina ate them for an hour straight and then complained of a stomachache. But, as the month went by, Laura noticed the supply of jelly beans dwindling more and more slowly while requests for other nutrient-packed snacks such as fruit, yogurt, crackers, and popcorn increased. Her daughter didn't ask for more jelly beans until two months later when she had a slumber party and her friends ate the rest of them.

This is not a dream; this can be a reality. Give your daughter a full supply of her favorite "forbidden" foods and do your best to ignore her eating behavior. Your daughter may eat more of the previously restricted foods for a while, but when she realizes that the jelly beans or chips or ice cream (or any other food) are no longer forbidden, she won't want them all the time and will start wanting other foods. When you legalize forbidden foods, they lose their magic. The same will happen with your eating behavior.

To begin the process of legitimizing *all* food choices:

- Inform your daughter that she can eat *anything* she wants.
- Make sure that her favorite foods are available in the house.
- Ask her to add some foods to the grocery list each week.
- Take her grocery shopping and have her choose some foods from each section: her favorite fruits and vegetables, her favorite cereal, her favorite cookies, etc.
- Keep your promise and let her eat *anything* she wants—even if it's Cap'n Crunch every morning. You can explain to her that other cereals will give more fiber or suggest that she have Cap'n Crunch every other day, but if she's hungry for it every day, let her have it

and provide some fruit, juice, and/or toast along with it so that her breakfast will be more nutritionally balanced.

Now, if your daughter is allergic to certain foods or has a medical condition that warrants her staying away from certain foods, you may have to find alternatives to her food requests that have similar tastes and consistencies. If she is allergic to milk products and says she wants ice cream, suggest sorbet or an ice pop. If she is diabetic and frequently requests high-sugar foods, find some artificially sweetened foods that are satisfying to her.

In every situation, when she's hungry, ask "What are you hungry for?" If she draws a blank and doesn't know, help her narrow down her options. Ask her if she wants something sweet, spicy, or salty; something hot, cold, or at room temperature; or something soft, chewy, or crunchy. If she still can't identify a specific food, it could be that her body really doesn't care—it just wants fuel, and probably just about anything will satisfy her. One mother used this opportunity to give her the most nutritious food in the house. "If it doesn't matter, I'll really pack in the nutrients."

Is Your Hunger Satisfied?

If it's chocolate she really wants, a pound of BBQed chicken won't satisfy her hunger. It it's BBQed chicken she wants, a pound of chocolate won't do the trick. When she eats exactly what she wants, her hunger is more easily satisfied with smaller amounts.

But only your daughter knows when her hunger is satisfied— not you or the amount on her plate. In order to make the decision to stop eating, she needs to know that there is an ample supply of the food she's eating and that she can have more later without judgment or criticism. She needs to know that her brother won't devour the rest of the pizza or you won't finish off the freshly picked blueberries. This prevents what I call the "Last Supper Syndrome" where we think we need to eat it all now because we don't know when we will get another chance. If she knows that there's plenty for later, she has no reason to overeat.

To help your daughter distinguish between satisfying her hunger and overeating:

- Have her hold up her fist and tell her that's the approximate size of her stomach—most of the time it won't take much food to fill her stomach and satisfy her, but sometimes it may take quite a bit of food.

- Recommend that she start with a smaller amount of food with the assurance that if she is still hungry, she can have more.

- As she is getting in the swing of knowing how much food satisfies her, while she's eating, ask her "Is your hunger satisfied?" (or "Is your hunger gone?" if she is younger). But don't go overboard with this question. If you ask her too often, she may feel pestered and start resenting the question.

By focusing on these three questions—Are you hungry? What are you hungry for? Is your hunger satisfied?—and responding to your daughter's answers, you may be concerned that you will have to shop every day and cook separate meals. Leave behind some of the myths about being a good mother: a meal doesn't have to be hot to be nutritious nor does it have to contain all the food groups. The *only* prerequisite is that you have a variety of foods around the house that your daughter can choose from or that you can offer. But nonetheless, you may have to set some limits. If she asks for fifty foods from the grocery store, you may have to tell her she can have ten. If you are in the car on the way home and she wants grapes, you don't have to search for the nearest produce stand. Tell her you have some grapes (or cantaloupe or other satisfying fruit) at home and will be there in a couple of minutes.

Some mothers are also concerned about the breakdown of the dinner meal because this approach may mean that the family won't always be eating together. But hasn't the family dinner meal already broken down over the years? We used to eat a leisurely, family-oriented dinner between 5 and 6 P.M. Now, with 87 percent of all single and 73 percent of all married mothers working,[4] fathers commuting, and kids having extracurricular activities after school, the rushed dinner meal is between 7 and 8 P.M.—and everyone is famished, tired, and irritable. On those days that everyone is home early, enjoy a relaxed, pleasurable meal, but on other later days, have an easy, lighter dinner at 7:30 P.M. or let your daughter eat earlier to meet her body's needs and set family time from 7 to 8 P.M. with a conversation hour, a game, or a book.

With your concerns put to rest, have fun with your new, healthy mother-daughter food relationship. Encourage your daughter to explore, discover, and experiment without judgment or consequences. *Self-discovery is a part of the learning process.*

In a professional article entitled "The Play Approach to Learning in the Context of Families and Schools: An Alternative Paradigm for Nutrition and Fitness Education in the 21st Century," the authors conclude that "merging the play approach to learning . . . will result in a generation of youth that laughs a little more, plays a little more, moves a little more, and finds joy in eating. . . ."[5] I couldn't agree more. The didactic, authoritarian approach to nutrition education hasn't worked very well.

DAUGHTER-FRIENDLY FOOD ADVICE

I understand the need to teach my daughter about her instinctive food needs, but don't I need to teach my daughter about good nutrition too?
—Cynthia, age 29

Nutrition education is important, but we need a new, nonthreatening, nonjudgmental method of teaching nutrition to our daughters, one that assists them in making food choices—not one that condemns them for making "bad" choices or praises them for making "good" choices.

The good food/bad food method of nutrition education has backfired. Focusing on the evils of fat, salt, sugar, and processed foods has not decreased dieting, disordered eating, or weight preoccupation. In fact, the opposite has been found to be true. Studies have shown that adolescent girls seek out nutrition knowledge in order to pursue the perfect diet and the perfect body.

In truth, your daughter may know more about the principles of healthy eating than you do. In a nationwide survey, only 77 percent of adults surveyed were familiar with the food groups, whereas

95 percent of adolescents were. In addition, 99 percent of adolescents understood the link between nutrition and health and 98 percent understood the importance of fruits and vegetables.[6] But as you may know all too well, understanding doesn't always translate to behavior changes.

So, how can you subtly veer your daughter toward a nutritious, balanced diet without causing increased food and weight preoccupation?

The Dietary Guidelines for Americans, introduced over fifteen years ago by the United States Department of Agriculture and the Department of Health and Human Services, have recently undergone a revision that I commend.[7] Acknowledging the growing problems associated with restrictive eating and weight preoccupation, they emphasize the importance of variety, balance, moderation, choice, food pleasure, and exercise. The new changes also put more focus on the total diet (vs. individual food choices), which will help your daughter understand that "diet" really means daily food intake and not caloric restriction—and that within the context of a balanced diet, *no* food is off limits.

1. Eat a **variety** of foods.

2. **Balance** the food you eat with **physical activity**—maintain or improve your weight.

3. **Choose** a diet with plenty of grain products, vegetables, and fruits.

4. **Choose** a diet low in fat, saturated fat, and cholesterol.

5. **Choose** a diet **moderate** in sugars.

6. **Choose** a diet **moderate** in salt and sodium.

7. If you drink alcohol, do so in **moderation.**

These guidelines, as well as similar guidelines issued by the American Heart Association and American Cancer Society, may be advising that we eat a diet (total daily food intake) with less fat to achieve the recommended fat intake of 30 percent of total calories, but they are *not* advising that we eliminate fat from our diets. We have misinterpreted the message to mean that any fat is bad, less is good, and none is great.

The reality, though, is that with an average of about 38 percent of our calories coming from fat, the typical adult and child are eating too much fat.[8] Of course, that's the average; some are consuming too much less—and others are consuming too much more. Because eating habits are initially set in childhood, studies have found that young children with a very high fat intake continue to have a high fat intake as they mature.

If you think that you and your daughter are eating too much fat, how can you moderate your fat intakes without going overboard?

1. **Provide a variety of foods with varying fat contents so that she has greater choice.** Stock up on such naturally low-fat snacks and cookies as pretzels, bagels, ginger snaps, popcorn cakes, flavored rice cakes, animal crackers, graham crackers, vanilla wafers, and fig bars.

2. **Trust her food needs.** My observation with adults holds true for children: when they listen and respond to their food needs, their fat intake automatically comes down to a moderate level. They no longer restrict and then overindulge, and their starch intake naturally increases because their bodies need more carbohydrates than fats. As you are waiting for your daughter's fat intake to come down naturally, the rest of these suggestions should give you the peace of mind that you are having a positive impact on moderating your daughter's fat intake.

3. **Make some changes in what she doesn't see.** For example:

   - Trim meats before cooking.
   - Buy leaner cuts of meat, such as London broil, flank steak, and pork tenderloin.
   - Buy leaner luncheon meats, such as ham, roast beef, and, of course, the old standbys turkey and chicken breast.
   - Offer occasional vegetarian meals to lend variety.
   - Prepare foods with less added fat.
   - Experiment with some lower-fat recipes—many dishes are un-

necessarily high in fat, and you can cut some fat out of the recipe without reducing flavor or satisfaction.

4. **Do a fat-free taste test and let *her* decide if she likes the fat-free or the regular versions.** Does your kitchen look like a fat-free zone? If that's all you offer and she doesn't find the fat-free foods satisfying, she'll search for satisfaction at school, at the store on the way home, or at a friend's house. Being a potato chip connoisseur myself, I have yet to find a tolerable nonfat chip. And the nonfat cheese—I'd rather not eat cheese at all!

One frustrated mother declared, "My daughter doesn't like any of the fat-free foods; all she likes is junk food and fast food." My interpretation of *junk* food is *just understand the needs of kids*. Sometimes their bodies need fat, sugar, and fast food to provide a concentrated source of calories for growth—and something fun to eat.

5. **Don't ban your daughter from fast food.** How can you not let your daughter go to McDonald's and have french fries? Don't you want some too? Fast food is a part of our culture—37 percent of Americans eat fast food eight or more times a month.[9] The Golden Arches don't have to be the entryway to "fat city." Here are a few fast food surprises:

- Most milkshakes are surprisingly low in fat, with a range of 13 to 20 percent of the calories derived from fat.

- Regular hamburgers usually have about 30 percent of the calories from fat—and are one of the lowest fat choices (along with the chicken breast sandwiches, unless they have a secret sauce).

- A regular order of french fries has 10 grams of fat; a super size has 26 grams of fat.

- Ordering ham or Canadian bacon on a pizza (instead of pepperoni or sausage) can cut the fat content in half.

- Despite the high consumption of fast food and "junk" food, adolescents' nutritional status is good.[10] These foods do provide nutrition, particularly protein, iron, vitamin B12, and riboflavin.

6. Watch out for food commercials. Researchers at the University of Minnesota viewed more than fifty hours of Saturday morning programming and counted about 1,000 food commercials: 500 were for candy, cookies, chips, and sugared foods and drinks, 300 were for high-sugar cereals.[11] *Not one was for fruits or vegetables.*

The Tufts University Diet and Nutrition newsletter took this information and figured out what a child's diet would be if she ate the foods advertised on Saturday morning TV—and compared it to the USDA's recommended food guide pyramid.[12]

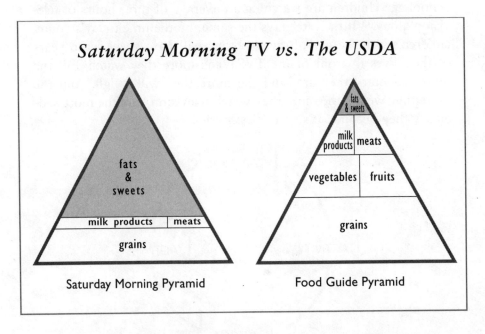

Saturday Morning TV vs. The USDA

Saturday Morning Pyramid

Food Guide Pyramid

If your daughter has an affinity for fat and sugar, food advertising may be partially to blame. You can't ban your daughter from watching television, but you can ask her if she is hungry, suggest other foods, and give her other nutrient-packed foods along with the Twinkies.

Through the power of suggestion, food commercials can trigger eating. But as we and our daughters become instinctive eaters, television's influence becomes less powerful. Of course, television has an impact not only on the behavior it potentially produces but also on the behavior it prevents.

DAUGHTER-FRIENDLY FITNESS ADVICE

I have two daughters. One watches TV all day and is overweight; the other is one of those fitness fanatics who works out every day.

—Jessica, age 41

School-age children are watching an average of three hours of television a day.[13] If the rate stays the same, by the time today's young children reach the age of seventy, they will have spent seven years of their lives in front of the TV.[14] The more they watch TV, the more sedentary they are, and the more they will weigh. And the more they weigh, the more they watch television, and the more sedentary they become. It's an endless cycle.

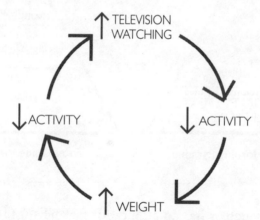

Television does more than contribute to a sedentary lifestyle. Researchers at Memphis State University found that watching television reduced metabolic rate in adolescent girls by 12 to 16 percent—which was a greater reduction in their metabolism than if they just sat on the couch and stared at a blank wall.[15] It's not yet clear why watching television slows down metabolism, but it may have to do with the mesmerizing effect of the screen, which causes a type of meditation state.

To boost our daughters' metabolisms, promote healthy weight loss, and improve their health, *we have to get them away from the tube and on the move!*

- The Massachusetts Governor's Committee on Physical Fitness and Sports reported that only 32% of our children had satisfactory levels of fitness (down from 43% in 1980).[16]

- When four- to seven-year-olds were asked what it takes to be healthy, 82% said eating the right foods—and only 17% said exercise.[17] Exercise needs to be the number-one answer, or at least tied for the number-one spot with healthy eating.

- Of 12,000 high school students studied in the Youth Risk Behavior Study, 52% of the female students were not enrolled in physical education classes.[18]

- Appearance is the primary motivation for exercise in young women, whereas fitness is the motivator for young men. In a survey of over 30,000 readers of *Psychology Today,* those women who valued fitness had better body images than those who valued appearance.[19] *Women can learn to value fitness too and use it as a powerful exercise motivator.*

If you instill the importance of regular physical activity for fitness, health, and enjoyment early on, research has shown that exercise will likely be an integral part of your daughter's lifestyle into adulthood.[20] In addition, by making exercise a part of *your* life, it will likely become a part of *her* life. A Boston University study found that a mother's level of activity correlates with that of her children. If she exercised, her children were *twice* as likely to exercise.[21]

So we need to model, support, and encourage an active lifestyle that is based on lifelong fitness, but as with nutrition education, we need to do it with a nonthreatening, middle-of-the-road approach so that our daughters neither underexercise nor overexercise. The world of fitness is filled with too many do's; instead let's focus on what you and your daughter *don't* have to do to get fit and enjoy all the wonderful benefits of exercise.

YOU *DO NOT* HAVE TO EXERCISE EVERY DAY

Women who maintain a comfortable weight are not exercise fanatics. To keep body fat at a healthy 25 percent, 86 percent of the women studied exercised only three to four times a week.[22] Exercising five, six, or seven days a week does not provide significant additional benefits. Incidentally, none of these women was dieting, and the most popular activity of all was walking.

YOU *DO NOT* HAVE TO RUN

You also do not have to rollerblade, go to step classes, do cross-training, or invest in today's most popular piece of fitness equipment—if you don't want to. But you do have to do an aerobic activity at a moderate intensity to derive the many physical benefits. Walking gives just as many benefits as any other form of aerobic exercise, but what's important is to choose one that you enjoy and then push yourself—but don't overdo it. If you do choose walking, take Harry Truman's advice. During his presidency, he recommended walking as if you have someplace important to go.

YOU *DO NOT* HAVE TO PUMP IRON

You don't have to bench press 150 pounds, you don't have to use the Nautilus-type equipment, you don't have to buy dumbbells (I've always wondered why they are called that), and you don't have to hire a personal trainer to "pump you up." Weight-lifting will tone, build muscle, and prevent some muscle and bone loss that occurs with aging, but it's not aerobic, so do it in addition to your walk or bike ride.

YOU *DO NOT* HAVE TO RELY ON MALE-FOCUSED RESEARCH

You have the right to a special exercise program that is designed for your female body. The traditional exercise guidelines are based on research using males as the study's subjects to determine how much they need to exercise for weight loss and improved cardiovascular fitness. But our bodies are different and deserve special attention with a female-oriented fitness program.

The reality is that women need to exercise 50 to 100 percent longer than men to get the same benefits. A study at the USDA Western Human Nutrition Research Center in San Francisco showed that women have to exercise forty-five to sixty minutes to get the same benefit as men exercising twenty-eight to thirty-five minutes.[23] This is why I strongly recommend a minimum of forty-five minutes—I want you to enjoy the benefits of exercising rather than feel frustrated and confused because your body isn't responding. Again "the more, the better" mentality doesn't work. Exercising over sixty minutes a session does not appear to provide significant additional benefits.

So, forty-five minutes of moderate activity three times a week is the answer for weight loss, improved health, and improved self-esteem. If your daughter is eleven years old or older, this is her exercise prescription too. If she is under eleven years old, a total of one hour of cumulative active play a day is recommended[24]—even if she is overweight.

BUT . . . MY DAUGHTER *IS* OVERWEIGHT

*My daughter is overweight, so don't I need to reduce her
fat intake and up her exercise more than the average
person?*
                                                    —*Donna, age 36*

Your overweight daughter does not need a special eating or exercise program and is entitled to make her own food and exercise decisions. When she decides when, what, and how much to eat, she will lose weight. In her groundbreaking work, Ellyn Satter (author of *How to Get Your Kids to Eat, But Not Too Much*) has proven that when parents of overweight kids back off, their children will eventually lose weight. If they are controlled and deprived, they will become food preoccupied and gain weight.

The instinctive eating approach works for weight loss! A program called Undieting at the University of Toronto found that positive changes in the diet mentality occured when an internally guided approach was used.[25] In just ten weeks, they found a:

- 36% increase in self-esteem
- 50% decrease in feelings of ineffectiveness
- 40% decrease in the drive for thinness
- 20% decrease in restrained eating

Once attitudes are adjusted and self-esteem is improved, weight loss will follow. Another recent study found that the nondiet approach resulted in a significant amount of weight loss that was maintained over the two-year period studied.[26] *The way to take weight off and keep it off is by staying off diets and by listening to your body's food needs.* And, of course, by exercising.

Many mothers have tried to encourage their overweight daughters to exercise and have concluded, "My daughter tried exercise and quit. She just doesn't want to exercise." Are you sure? A recent survey revealed that 80 percent of the adolescents expressed a desire to be more physically fit.[27] Maybe she doesn't want to exercise because she feels uncomfortable in an aerobics class or at the health club. One daughter shared with me, "They were all in these skimpy leotards, all skinny, and all looked like they could be aerobics instructors. I was the only one overweight." Make your daughter feel as comfortable as possible while exercising—buy or rent some aerobic videos so she can exercise in the house, go for a walk with her, or do some research to find a class that caters to all shape and sizes.

If your daughter is overweight:

- Exercise is vital. If she is eleven years or older, forty-five minutes three times a week is all she needs.
- Dieting is futile (but you already know that).
- Help her set realistic goals by taking genetics and the realities of the

pear-shaped female body into consideration. As soon as she hits puberty, the fat in her buttocks, hips, and thighs is more resistant to weight loss. Inform her that fat in her upper body will be easier to lose than fat in her lower body. As one daughter surmised, "You mean it's easier to lose fat in my gut than in my butt?" Well, yes. That's one way of saying it.

- Ask the three key questions—Are you hungry? What are you hungry for? Is your hunger satisfied?—and give your daughter food autonomy. Restricting her or telling her what she's doing wrong isn't helpful, it's hurtful.

To fully employ these suggestions, you may have to confront some of your own biases and misconceptions about being overweight. For example:

- Baby fat is *not* obesity; it's necessary. Young children need some extra body fat for growth and development.

- An overweight child will *not* necessarily become an overweight adult. Most studies have found a minimal relationship between obesity in childhood and obesity in adulthood.[28]

- Most overweight children do *not* overeat. In fact, studies have shown that they consume the same or less fat, sugar, and calories as slender kids.[29]

Analyze your own attitudes and biases about being overweight—you may be projecting your own weight issues on to your daughter. Treat her as a separate person and trust her eating instincts.

If you encourage the instinctive eating approach but your daughter still wants to diet, let her make the decision. With your new knowledge about the dangers of dieting, you may be tempted to forbid dieting—which may make her want to diet all the more. Dieting may be a way to resist your control or to guarantee your control. If she sees that you are indifferent, the fad will pass. But if you draw attention to dieting and she continues, she may be headed down the path to an eating disorder.

BUT . . . MY DAUGHTER *HAS* AN EATING DISORDER

My daughter was overweight, then she started dieting and it took over her life. Now she weighs ninety-six pounds and is anorexic. What can I do to help her?

—*Serena, age 47*

If your daughter has an eating disorder—anorexia, bulimia, or compulsive overeating—or an exercise disorder, she and you need more than this book to foster a healthy mother-daughter food relationship. Her unhealthy eating habits are a symptom of a greater underlying psychological problem—and that problem needs to be identified and treated. Although the instinctive eating approach is the solution from a behavioral standpoint, she needs to be psychologically ready for it. But you *can* help her now!

1. **Know the signs of an eating disorder** so that you can identify whether your daughter needs help or not—and whether you are in denial or not. Parents often are.

   - Is she regularly skipping or avoiding meals?
   - Is she sneaking food? Do you find large amounts of food missing?
   - Does she routinely visit the bathroom after eating?
   - Is she talking about food and her weight all the time?
   - Is she exercising excessively?
   - Does she have frequent and significant weight fluctuations?

   If you have any doubt as to whether your daughter has an eating disorder, contact an eating disorders specialist and share your concerns.

2. **Speak up.** If you think your daughter has an eating disorder, without accusing her, tell her that you are concerned and base your comments on your observations. For example, say:

- "Lately I've noticed that you are eating only one meal a day, and I'm concerned about you."

- "I've often smelled vomit in the bathroom after you've been in there, and I want to help you."

- "I'm aware that you're exercising at least two hours a day, and often at the expense of homework, social activities, and family functions."

3. **Find a licensed therapist** who has experience treating eating disorders (not all therapists do) and uses a multidisciplinary approach with a physician, psychiatrist, and nutritionist. Interview the therapist and some other members of the team to make sure they are the right people for your daughter *and* you to work with. Be a part of her therapy as recommended by her therapist and make it a priority to have your daughter regularly meet with her or him. Recognize that you too may need some counseling to take care of yourself.

4. **Educate yourself about eating disorders** by reading books and newsletters and contact support groups and organizations. (A listing is provided at the end of the book.)

5. **Be a part of your daughter's recovery** in a way that's appropriate for her.

- Ask her how she wants you to be involved.
- Do not monitor her progress verbally; don't make food an issue.
- Keep your promises; foster a sense of trust.

6. **Don't carry the guilt** that you are solely responsible for her eating disorder. Acknowledge how you may have influenced her eating behavior, apologize to her, and move on. Guilt will not help her—love and caring will.

7. **Admit your own limitations,** let her know that you are not perfect.

8. **Be patient.** Part of her needs the eating disorder, so support her until she doesn't need it any longer.

You can do all this—and more—but there is a world out there perpetuating the culture of dieting, the pursuit of thinness, and the eventual development of eating disorders. Despite the world's reinforcement of negative behaviors, an experienced therapist can help your daughter deal with it and put it into perspective. But eating disordered or not, certain individuals may be working against your efforts.

OTHER THAN MOTHER: WHO ELSE IS INFLUENCING YOUR DAUGHTER?

> *My mother and father never make any negative comments about my body. I have an older sister who does that for me. She tells me that my butt is so big she could have a picnic on it.*
>
> *—Kimberly, age 14*

You are the primary source of nutrition information for your daughter, but extended family, peers, and other adults such as caregivers, teachers, coaches, and doctors also shape your daughter's food and body relationship. It's vital to identify these people and balance their influence. Talk to them and talk to your daughter about them.

Here are some examples of how other individuals have affected young, impressionable women—and what can be done to put their influences in perspective.

SIBLING WEIGHT RIVALRY

"My sister is always called the 'adorably petite' one; I am always called the 'smart' one. I've grown up thinking that I am the ugliest thing on the planet because I have a bigger bone structure than my sister. I slouch to make my body look smaller, diet to make my body shrink, and am in an unspoken weight-loss competition with her."

If you have two or more daughters, treat them equally. If one is overweight and one is at a comfortable weight, trust both of their eating instincts. Sit them down for a talk and discuss how different genes in their family tree have influenced their body shapes and how they both can accept and respect their bodies.

PEER PRESSURE

"My friend Missy taught me everything I ever wanted to know about dieting—and I wasn't afraid to ask. She read every book and magazine article on the subject and bought every weight-loss gadget, drink, and pill that came on the market. Her family moved five years ago, but she left a pair of her size-four jeans as my weight-loss incentive. I remember her saying 'The day you fit into these jeans will be the happiest day of your life.' I still have the jeans to remind me that I have yet to find happiness."

Peers can be the most influential. If your daughter has a friend who is doing a juice fast to clean out her colon and she wants to do it too, you can give her accurate information and let her know that a fast will slow down her metabolism and activate her fat cells—then leave the decision up to her. If you tell her that she can't do it, she may rebel and definitely fast. In addition, forbidding her doesn't solve the problem, it adds another one. You are forcing her to choose between you and her friend.

FATHERLY INFLUENCE

"My dad used to have me draw stick figures because that's what he wanted me to look like. Now he weighs me every morning before school, tells me that boys prefer thin girls, and bribes me to lose weight with money and clothes. When my weight is down, he showers me with love and affection; when my weight is up, he gives me the silent treatment and doesn't talk to me for days."

Most fathers are not as abusive as this example, but they may make comments or encourage negative behaviors that will affect their daughters for the rest of their lives. A father's reaction to his daughter's changing body during adolescence influences her self-esteem and body image. It's important that you and her father (whether you are married to him or not) are consistent, giving the same messages about eating and exercising and the same guidance on body acceptance and self-esteem. If it's impossible to reach an agreement with her father, do your best to balance his negative influence by complimenting all of your daughter's qualities (including talents and skills) and encouraging her to acknowledge her own strengths.

I don't want to leave you with the impression that fathers are responsible for their daughters' poor body image and disordered eating behavior. A few may be, but most fathers positively affect their daughters' self-esteem through unconditional love, infinite pride, and daily compliments.

MOTHER'S HELPERS:
AUNTS, GRANDMOTHERS, CAREGIVERS

"My aunt comes to stay with us once a year when my mom and dad go on vacation. I remember last year, she looked at me with a skeptical eye and told me that she was going to get rid of my baby fat. She threw away all the food in the house and stocked the refrigerator with grapefruit and cottage cheese. She also had an ample supply of prescription diet pills and had me taking four a day. Both she and I would be up most of the night because we couldn't sleep from the amphetamines. She was so pleased that I had lost eight pounds in a week. Of course, when she left, she took her diet pills with her and I quickly gained ten pounds, but she was responsible for triggering my weight preoccupation and dieting obsession."

Just because they are family doesn't give them permission to negatively influence your daughter. Firmly ask that they cooperate with your wishes. They may disagree with what you are doing, but ultimately they too may benefit from the instinctive eating approach. Also, tell your daughter to be as specific as possible with her food requests, saying, for example, "I'm hungry and I'd like a piece of cheese, please" or "I'm not hungry right now, but maybe I'll have something later."

COACHES, AEROBICS INSTRUCTORS, AND FITNESS GURUS

"My high school gymnastics coach is my dieting mentor. She has an incredibly thin body, and we sit and talk for hours about how I can have a body just like hers. She takes our body measurements once a week and weighs us at every practice. If our weights are up, we have to practice an extra hour every day until she's satisfied with the numbers on the scale."

Talk to your daughter's coaches and instructors and set some "rules" on what they can and can't do. Depending on the situation, you may also have to talk to the school board.

DOCTORS, DENTISTS, AND MEDICAL CHIEFS

"I have a seven-year-old daughter. When we went for her last doctor's appointment, he showed her the growth charts and said, 'See, you're at the fiftieth percentile for height and the eighty-fifth percentile for weight. Now, do you think you have a weight problem, Kelly?' I was so angry with him. I immediately said, 'NO, we do not have a weight problem!' but the comment stuck with my daughter. I see her getting on the scale and telling her friends that her doctor told her she was too fat and she needed to lose weight."

You may have to have a talk with her doctor and/or find a new pediatrician. Interview them and make sure their eating and weight philosophies coincide with your new instinctive approach to eating.

Most important, for all outside influences and people, provide an environment where your daughter can share her feelings and talk to you. Help her realize that she is not alone (you have experienced these influences too), she does have options, and *she* is the decision maker. She can set limits with these people, ask them not to do certain things, and ask them to support her efforts in a way that's right for her. She can also seek out individuals who are instinctive eaters and will reinforce her and your efforts.

By balancing these other influences, trusting your own eating instincts, and teaching your daughter to trust hers, you will evoke the rebirth of your healthy mother-daughter food relationship. Now, with the final chapter, to fully transform the generation trap of disordered eating into a generational triumph of instinctive eating, you will focus on mending the food relationship you have with your own mother—and guarantee a healthy legacy for you, your mother, your daughter, and future generations of women.

CHAPTER EIGHT

LIKE MOTHER, LIKE DAUGHTER: FROM GENERATION TRAP TO GENERATION TRIUMPH

*Y*ou, *your mother,* and your daughter are having dinner at your favorite restaurant. In the past, all three of you used to order the grilled chicken breast salad without even glancing at the menu. But tonight you are carefully analyzing the selections to choose exactly what you want. The waiter comes to your table to take your order, and you say, "I'll have the sautéed mushroom appetizer to start and the lobster ravioli appetizer as my main dish." Your mother looks at you, laughs, and tells the waiter she'll have the same, except in the opposite order. Now it's your teenage daughter's turn to order, and she says, "I'll have the lobster ravioli appetizer too, but I'll start with the chocolate torte as my first course." The waiter gives her a quizzical look, shrugs his shoulders, and walks away.

If restaurants are finally getting used to our low-fat requests, they had better prepare themselves for yet another change in restaurant etiquette. As more and more of us break out of the trap of disordered eating and dieting, the order of the menu will become meaningless. We will not always be eating the appetizer first, main dish next, and dessert last. Instead, we may decide to start with a dessert, or end the meal with soup, or order two appetizers instead of a main course. With our bodies directing our food needs, *anything* is possible.

And not only restaurants will experience the impact of this new pattern of eating. Grocery stores, college cafeterias, food caterers, health spas, food companies, nutrition education classes, bookstores, snack bars, and coffee shops will all be affected by the new way women buy and eat food. We are making changes that will shape business, industry, education, society—and the typical day in America. As we make the triumphant personal transformation to instinctive eating, all those involved in either the world of marketing and preparing food or that of physical fitness will have no choice but to change with us. The habits and attitudes of disordered eaters will no longer prevail because they are worlds apart from this new breed of instinctive eaters.

A Disordered Eater	An Instinctive Eater
diets	doesn't think about dieting
ignores her hunger signals	responds to hunger signals
eats for emotional nourishment	eats for physical nourishment
restricts foods	permits all foods
fights food cravings	welcomes food cravings
denies herself food pleasure	seeks food pleasure
undereats and/or overeats	eats to satisfy hunger
follows society's eating rules	follows her body's eating rules
is unaware of her food needs	is in tune with her food needs
fights her body	respects her body
focuses on appearance	focuses on self-acceptance
experiences weight fluctuations	maintains a comfortable weight

You and your daughter are already making this vital transformation by establishing a healthy mother-daughter food relationship. But to fully achieve the reversal of the disordered eating legacy, an essential third person needs to be included: *your mother.* You need to come to peace with her legacy and to recognize how you may be passing any or all of it on to your daughter. Much of the guidance in this book has been directed toward healing the food relationship you have with your daughter, but to benefit your entire family, it's equally important to develop a healthier food relationship with your mother as well.

Depending on the dynamics of your current situation with your mother, this new food and body relationship may take a variety of different forms: It may mean that you both work together to become instinctive eaters; it may mean healing yourself first and then helping her break free from the disordered eating trap; it may mean reaching an agreement where she refrains from certain behaviors or comments; or it may mean learning independent coping skills to change the way *you* react to your mother's influence.

Whatever form your healthier adult mother-daughter food relationship takes, you must first try to gain insight into the reasons behind your mother's actions, attitudes, and comments—and begin the process of transforming blame to understanding.

FROM MOTHER BLAMING TO MOTHER RECLAIMING

When my mother and I finally talked about our weight and food issues, I realized the great pressure she felt to make my body acceptable.

—*Jody, age 41*

Jody had spent the last twenty-five years blaming her mother for her eating disorder. Her mother was bulimic and taught Jody how to self-induce vomiting at age thirteen. "One day we were driving in the car and she told me that my father (her ex-husband) wouldn't make love to her unless she weighed 120 pounds or less. All of a sudden, it hit me; I realized bulimia was her survival strategy, and she thought that I also needed it for future male relationships."

Whether your mother directly initiated an eating disorder or indirectly influenced your unhealthy eating habits and poor body image, taking the time to understand the context of her influence can help you move beyond blame and begin healing the relationship. This is a necessary step because harboring blame paralyzes change, keeps us trapped in disordered eating, causes feelings of guilt, and distracts attention from the cultural and personal issues that your mother was dealing with at the time. In *Feminist Perspectives on Eating Disorders,* Judith Rabinor described the paralyzing cycle when she wrote, "These feelings of blame and guilt produce and reinforce feelings of helplessness and powerlessness in mother and daughter alike, impairing the ability to grow."[1]

To break out of the cycle and establish a foundation of strength for your adult mother-daughter food relationship—and your personal instinctive eating journey—follow these steps:

REPHRASE BLAMING STATEMENTS TO QUESTIONS THAT ENCOURAGE UNDERSTANDING

What aspects of your unhealthy relationship with food and your body do you blame on your mother? With this question, some of my clients have wanted to go on for hours, blaming practically every aspect of their food and weight preoccupation on their mothers. I have included the three most common blaming statements given by daughters that I have interviewed. One or all of these may apply to your own mother-daughter food relationship, but what's most important is that you turn the statements into questions and begin the process of understanding your mother through revealing answers. To stimulate thought, I have provided a few sample answers for each question, but I encourage you to directly ask your mother "Why?" If that's too uncomfortable for you to do right now, you may be able to answer these questions yourself through the knowledge of your mother's past.

Blaming Statements	Rephrased Questions	Sample Answers
My mother overfed me.	Why did my mother overfeed me?	Food was her symbol of love. She experienced starvation. She thought fat was healthy.
My mother restricted my intake of fat and sugar.	Why did my mother restrict my intake of fat and sugar?	She was concerned about my health. Heart disease runs in my family. She was a restrained eater.
My mother encouraged me to diet.	Why did my mother encourage me to diet?	She dieted all of her life. She was trying to make sure I didn't inherit her obesity. She wanted me to be happy and successful.

After going through this process of rephrasing the statements into questions, one of my clients concluded, "Even though my mother controlled my eating habits and encouraged me to diet, she really isn't to blame; the dieting culture is to blame. My mother was affected by the same social pressures that I am." Most of my clients come to the same conclusion, and they realize that blaming their mothers keeps them from taking responsibility for their own lives. Be honest with yourself and separate her influence from your own issues.

If your mother has died, coming to this conclusion and moving beyond the blame may happen automatically. An analysis of my focus groups revealed that motherless daughters found little fault in the influence that their mothers had on their eating because they had already come to a deeper understanding of their mothers' behavior. When asked, "Did your mother ever put you on a diet?" a common response was "Well, yes, but she didn't know any better because everyone was dieting. However, she also taught me how to eat a balanced diet and why exercise was important." When left with only the memories of their mothers, my focus group participants chose to reflect more on the positive influences than the negative. If you are fortunate enough to still have your mother in your life, spend some time reflecting on the positives.

AFFIRM THE POSITIVE ASPECTS OF YOUR MOTHER-DAUGHTER FOOD RELATIONSHIP

I have not yet come across a daughter who did not have at least one positive recollection of her mother's influence on her eating behavior. Even Jody, whose mother taught her how to vomit, acknowledged that her mother also taught her that snacking was important throughout the day.

What positive influence did your mother have on your eating habits and body image? As you are contemplating your own answers, here are some my clients had to this question:

- "My mother taught me that round hips were beautiful."
- "My mother ate a wide variety of foods and always had everything from fruit to fudge available."
- "My mother was way ahead of her time and always made sure that we had whole-grain bread, fresh produce, and vegetarian dishes a couple of times a week."
- "Through her dieting failures, my mother indirectly taught me not to diet."

Affirming the positive aspects of your mother-daughter food relationship also means identifying enjoyable eating experiences, memorable rituals, and family traditions. What parts of your mother-daughter food relationship did you or do you enjoy?

- "Going out for our monthly dinners."
- "Being welcomed home with my favorite childhood dinner."
- "Spending the night before Thanksgiving preparing the feast, setting the table, and drinking wine together."

- "Making an authentic Greek meal with family recipes that have been passed down for generations."

Don't let the positive influences get buried beneath the negatives. Affirm other positive aspects of your mother-daughter relationship that have nothing to do with food, acknowledge the wisdom your mother passed on to you, reclaim your family traditions and ethnic dishes, and appreciate the pleasures of your mother-daughter food relationship. By doing so, you may find that your feelings toward your mother change: you may feel less anger, more empathy, and more joy.

EXPRESS YOUR FEELINGS

Depending on your relationship with your mother, expression of your feelings may vary. You may choose to talk to your mother directly, write her a letter that you never send, vocalize your feelings by talking to a friend or a therapist, or keep a journal of your feelings. Just don't keep them buried inside. An inability to express anger stunts healing, but so does dwelling on the anger. *Express your feelings, let go of them, and move on.* While this is not easy to do, it is an essential part of your healthy eating maturation process.

Opening the lines of emotional communication can bring you closer together. In a recent survey of over 1,000 daughters, 60 percent reported that they felt very close to their mothers. Although more than half of the daughters said they wanted to change something in their relationship with their mothers, the most common response was a change in geography, wishing that they lived closer to their mothers.[2]

FIND THE BALANCE BETWEEN CLOSENESS AND SEPARATION

A daughter's struggle between closeness and separation has been so extensively researched that special terms, matridentity and matrophobia, are now used to describe this internal conflict. *Matridentity* is the strong need to identify with our mothers and remain connected. *Matrophobia,* a term coined by Adrienne Rich, is our some-times consuming fear of becoming just like her.[3]

From my interviews with women, I found that those who con-tinue to struggle with the conflicting issues of closeness and sepa-ration were more likely to connect unconsciously with their mothers' food and weight issues. Sue was trying to separate from her mother geographically and emotionally; she moved away and seldom visited or talked with her mother on the phone. Then one day, sitting on the couch in my office, she told me about her experience in a de-partment store dressing room. "I was trying on an outfit, looked in the mirror, and saw my mother's behind. I've spent most of my life trying to be the opposite of my mother, but despite my efforts, I have become just like her anyway, butt and all." As she struggled to disassociate from her mother physically and emotionally, Sue un-consciously fulfilled the strong need to identify with her mother by weighing as much as she did. *Sometimes, the more phobic we are of becoming our mothers, the more likely we are to become them.*

We don't have to choose between matrophobia or matridentity as much as redefine our connection to our mothers and find the right balance between individuation and closeness. So I propose a third term, *matribalance,* that will help us create and maintain a healthy mother-daughter food and body relationship.

Thankfully, I have already achieved matribalance. I connect with my mother in many ways: we have similar personalities and almost identical body shapes. I take much pride in my closeness to her, but I am also thankful for the balance defined through sepa-ration. I have reached this balance in many ways, but my separation from my mother is particularly evident in our differing attitudes toward cooking—I have matrophobic tendencies in the kitchen.

In addition to her many other work and family activities, I've watched my mother forever cooking, cleaning, and shopping. Most of her time at home is spent *in the kitchen;* most of mine is spent *in my home office.* She goes grocery shopping almost every day; I try to limit it to once a month. She experiments with new recipes; I only cook pizza in three different ways—small, medium, and large. She has often asked "Where have I gone wrong as a mother?" Of course, she did nothing wrong—it was my choice to pursue another path from hers as homemaker.

She still occasionally starts a phone conversation by telling me of a new dish that she made last night, and I usually have to cut her off in midsentence to remind her which daughter she is talking to. And she still says that she's determined to teach me how to cook—someday. Let it go, Mom. It's my balance with separation and my rejection of the traditional female role you sometimes symbolize. It's also a sign of my independent, rebellious nature, which, even if I wanted to try my skill at cooking someday, would keep me out of the kitchen.

ACKNOWLEDGE YOUR CONTRIBUTION TO AN UNHEALTHY MOTHER-DAUGHTER FOOD RELATIONSHIP

How are you contributing to an unhealthy mother-daughter food relationship? How are you preventing its transformation to a healthier one?

Our actions, attitudes, habits, and weight can send varying messages to our mothers. For example, my stubborn culinary indifference tells my mother that she can't control me in the kitchen, no matter how hard she tries. What do your eating habits and/or body weight say to your mother?

- "I have perfect eating habits so I'm in control of my life and don't need you."

- "I have unhealthy eating habits so I'm out of control with my life and still need you."

- "I'm overweight and have extra layers of fat to protect me so you don't need to worry about me."

- "I'm overweight and not taking care of myself so you still have to worry about me."

- "I'm overweight because I want to upset you."

- "I'm underweight because I want to upset you."

- "I'm underweight, disciplined, self-confident, and socially accepted so I can take care of myself."

- "I'm underweight and weak so I can't take care of myself."

It takes two to form a food relationship. Acknowledge your role as well as your mother's and go on to claim a healthier future.

ACCEPT RESPONSIBILITY FOR YOUR OWN RELATIONSHIP WITH FOOD

No matter how your mother might have influenced your eating behavior during childhood, *you* are responsible for your own relationship with food. Regardless of how your mother tries to influence you today, *you* are responsible for your own food decisions and how you respond to her influence.

What happens when you go home for a visit? Does your mother still overfeed you? Cook you diet meals? Comment on your weight? Many of my clients are tentative about returning home because as soon as they walk in the door, they say that they "become ten years old again."

When one of my clients, Renee, got an invitation to a family reunion, she considered declining. "I've been listening to my body and thought that I was over my food and weight preoccupations, but this invitation sent me into a frenzy. We haven't all been together for over ten years, and my Aunt Paula will definitely be there. She's the one who always said to me 'Your thighs look like they have gotten bigger, dear.' And when my mother and Aunt Paula get together, all they talk about is who gained weight, who lost weight, who shouldn't be eating dessert, and who should be dieting. I don't think I can handle it."

Renee eventually decided that she could handle it. Together, we went through the steps outlined in this section and prepared her for the reunion weekend. She understood that her aunt's and mother's comments were a projection of their own weight preoccupations and instead focused on the positive aspects of lively, delicious Italian meals with much laughter and acknowledged that she would only make the situation worse by not speaking up and taking care of herself.

When Renee returned from the family reunion, she excitedly reported on the positive outcome. "I exercised every other day, made my own food decisions, and instead of cowering at their comments, I stood up for myself. When as I predicted my aunt Paula said 'Your thighs look like they have gotten bigger, dear,' I said, 'Thanks for noticing, Aunt Paula. My muscles are really developing from my walking program, and I love their increased strength.' When my mother said 'You really shouldn't be eating dessert' I said, 'Oh, but I should because my body needs dessert right now, and I'm letting my body make my food decisions.' The best part was when my mother and aunt asked if I was on some kind of new diet, and I had the opportunity to tell them all about my instinctive eating program. We talked for hours, and now they're reconsidering dieting."

REVERSED ROLES: DAUGHTERS HELPING MOTHERS

> *My daughter has made a huge difference in my life over the past year. I entered menopause, started gaining weight, and proceeded to try one diet after another. She helped me start walking, walked with me, and encouraged me to stick with an exercise program.*
>
> —Barbara, age 53

As you are becoming an instinctive eater and reclaiming your healthier adult mother-daughter food relationship, you may find yourself wanting to help your mother and/or your mother turning to you for weight loss, health, and nutrition advice.

But, just as you are not responsible for your daughter's eating habits, you are also *not* responsible for your mother's eating habits and health. You can, however:

- tell her that you care
- ask her if and how she wants you to be involved (she may not want your help)
- follow through with her requests

Your mother may be quite receptive to your assistance. Women over the age of sixty have made the most positive changes in their lifestyle. They consume the most fruits and vegetables and are more likely to have made exercise a part of their lives.[4] They are also eager for medical information and are one of the highest users of libraries and other sources of health information. You can help to educate your mother without taking responsibility for her health—but only if she agrees to your help.

- **You can help put your mother's diet mentality in perspective.** If your mother calls saying that she gained six pounds overnight, you can explain to her that it is probably water weight because it's impossible to gain six pounds in twelve hours. (It would take at least 21,000 extra calories to gain six pounds!) At her request, you can also go over to her house and support her efforts to throw the scale in the garbage.

- **You can help your mother stop dieting.** If your mother is a professional dieter, you can share your new knowledge of the devastating effects of dieting on fat and muscle metabolism and encourage her to give the instinctive eating approach a try with your support. But if she decides to continue dieting, you can continue to be an instinctive eating role model for her—and hope that, someday, she may reconsider.

- **You can help your mother lose excess weight.** As a concerned daughter, you need to understand that even a moderate weight loss of 5 to 10 percent will significantly improve her health and decrease her risk of disease.[5] Losing too much weight may be unhealthy because carrying some extra reserves as she enters her seventies and eighties will actually increase her longevity.[6] Help her set realistic goals that are based on her age, menopausal changes, genetics, and optimal health—and, most important, help her with an exercise program.

- **You can help your mother make exercise a part of her life.** If your mother is sedentary, *any* movement is beneficial. If your mother is already exercising, you can help her tailor her exercise program to get the most benefits for weight loss and disease prevention. At every age, forty-five minutes three times a week will provide all the aerobic benefits needed. One study showed that after just ten weeks of aerobic exercise, women in their eighties and nineties doubled their leg muscle strength, walked 12 percent faster, and climbed stairs 30 percent easier.[7] To ensure maximum benefits, adding strength training will build bone and muscle and prevent the loss of these tissues that occurs with aging. Investigate exercise classes for older individuals, walk with her three times a week, or help her choose exercise equipment.

- **You can help your mother improve her overall health.** If your mother has high blood cholesterol, high blood pressure, and/or other health problems, you can tell her that you care about her and ask her how you can help. Can you buy her some books on diet and heart disease, enroll in a low-fat cooking class together, join her for walks, or go to the doctor's with her?

- **You can help your mother take care of her needs.** If your mother has been busy taking care of everyone else's needs, she may be forgetting about her own. This was the case with Rachel's mother. "My mother had five children, then, when we were out of the house, she cared for her dying parents. Now she's accepted the position of baby-sitter for her seven grandchildren, but she is starting to feel the effects of growing older and not taking care of herself all these years." Free up her time, designate "pampering" days to spend together, and help her feel comfortable taking time for herself.

Fulfilling the reversed role of helping your mother doesn't mean making sure that she becomes the healthiest woman on the planet. It means assisting your mother in ways that fit her personality, goals, and lifestyle. As you are providing mother-friendly food advice, you may also find yourself helping your father establish a healthier lifestyle. But father-friendly food advice will take an entirely different form because men approach weight loss, eating, and exercise differently than women. Maybe it's time to do some gender comparisons.

LIKE MOTHER, UNLIKE FATHER: GENERATIONS OF GENDER DIFFERENCES

My daddy eats and my mommy diets.

—Amy, age 7

This seven-year-old's observation of her mother's and father's eating behavior is simple yet precise. Men are less likely to want to try to lose weight and, therefore, less likely to diet and become disordered eaters. As you are reading this:

- Almost twice as many women as men are dieting.[8]

- Ten times as many women as men have an eating disorder.[9]

- More men (at least of those surveyed) want to gain weight rather than lose weight.[10]

Although some recent studies have shown that the incidence of eating disorders and body dissatisfaction is on the rise in young men, the majority are much less weight preoccupied compared to women. Many reasons exist for these gender differences, but the predominant one is the absence of a universally accepted ideal male body. When I asked my husband, "Is there an ideal body for men?" he contemplated the question for a moment then answered, "Not really. There is a V-shaped body with large muscular shoulders and a tapered waist, but most men disregard the Arnold Schwarzenegger-like image. We know it's unrealistic, and we don't compare ourselves to it so it doesn't affect our self-esteem."

My husband's attitude typifies that of most men. All studies have shown that weight is toward the bottom of the list of male self-esteem determinants. Men are more likely to base their self-worth on talents, accomplishments, and physical capabilities, not on appearance. Unlike thin women, thin men are not necessarily viewed as more attractive, successful, or popular. And unlike overweight women, overweight men are not as jeopardized in their marital, career, or financial success. As Ambrose Bierce wrote almost 100 years ago, "To men, a man is but a mind, who cares what face he carries or what form he wears, but a woman's body is the woman."[11] This holds true today and explains the vast differences in men's and women's dieting behaviors.

Fewer men diet because fewer men feel the need to diet to improve their body image. And when they do diet, they have better results. They lose twice as much weight, twice as quickly, and are twice as likely to keep it off. Men carry more muscle mass, have faster metabolisms, and are born with the fat-burning machinery to lose weight quickly and efficiently. It may not seem fair, but it's a medical fact.

Men are also more methodical and less emotional about weight loss. They identify the problem, choose the solution, and lose the weight. If they don't lose weight or if they regain it quickly after the diet, they do not view the diet failure as a personal failure. As one adult daughter reflected on the men in her life, "All of them—my father, husband, brothers, and sons—have never beaten themselves up over a diet failure. They don't worry about it, and they certainly don't waste any precious time, energy, or brain space obsessing about their bodies."

Think about it: Have you ever heard a man comment "I feel so fat today"? Have you seen men going through their closets in search of the perfect slimming outfit only to conclude that they have nothing to wear? Have you ever witnessed them talking to their male friends about how much weight they hope to lose on their new diet?

Probably not, but you may have seen them slap their stomachs and say that it's time to lose weight, then confidently go about their day without a second thought about it.

Just as daughters follow in their mothers' dieting and disordered eating footsteps, sons follow in their fathers' nondieting and higher self-esteem footsteps. The American Association of University Women study revealed that twice as many boys as girls rated their talents as what they liked best about themselves—and that twice as many girls as boys rated a body part as what they liked best about themselves.[12] Young girls base their self-esteem on how their bodies look, boys on what their bodies can do. Young boys want their bodies to get bigger and young girls want their bodies to get smaller. Young boys want to take up more space and young girls want to take up less. Because of these gender differences, by age thirteen, 80 percent of the girls have dieted, but only 10 percent of the boys have.[13] And by age eighteen, women desire to be at 87 percent of their recommended weights, men at 101 percent of their recommended weights.[14]

I do marvel at times at men's strong self-esteem regardless of their weight and wish that women too could separate who they are from what they weigh. Perhaps we can learn from the men in our lives, especially since fathers and husbands are starting to play a bigger role in parenting. The U.S. Department of Labor Statistics recently reported that more than 250,000 fathers are now at home raising their children.[15] And those who are not the single or at-home parent express the desire to spend more time with their families. The *Men's Life* survey found that 63 percent of the men under thirty-five considered family time a top priority.[16] As this trend in increased paternal involvement continues, fathers will have a greater opportunity to help model body acceptance for their daughters as well as the self-esteem benefits of physical capabilities, talents, and other accomplishments.

Fathers and other male figures can have a positive impact on young women today and in the future, but nothing takes the place of female friendships in your and your daughter's life. Women receive much personal satisfaction from the female community, and as studies have shown, men are more oriented to individualization whereas women are more oriented to socialization.

NONBIOLOGICAL MOTHERS: THE IMPORTANCE OF FEMALE COMMUNITY

> *My friends and I have all said farewell to dieting, and I feel confident that my daughter's exposure to successful, nondieting women will help balance the outside pressure to be unnaturally thin.*
>
> —Mary Pat, age 40

As I discussed in the previous chapter, a few individuals may have a negative influence on your daughter's relationship with food, but the majority of the women in your daughter's life can have a powerful, positive impact. They can model nondieting behavior, show that they too have been affected by society's pressure for thinness and the culture of dieting, and share how in the midst of these pressures they have accepted their bodies.

The power of female camaraderie, support, and nurturance is a wonderful force to witness. One evident example is in the African American community where a number of women share the responsibilities of mothering, not just the mother. The famous African proverb "It takes a village to raise a child" continues to have meaning today as grandmothers, sisters, older siblings, and friends form a circle of mothers who give strength to a young woman's definition of womanhood. And this support and strength is one of the primary reasons why black women have a lower incidence of dieting, disordered eating, and eating disorders—and a more positive body image.

For all ethnic groups, *social support is vital*—for validation, self-esteem, and the guidance of female wisdom. This social support comes from family, extended family, stepmothers, stepsisters, friends, female-oriented organizations, the work environment, support groups, church groups, school groups, political groups, exercise groups, women's groups, book groups, and potentially any woman in your community.

Name at least five women in your female community who are important to you and your sense of self. Have your daughter do the same. You may find that some of the same names appear on both your lists.

5 Important Women in Your Life	5 Important Women in Your Daughter's Life
1._____	1._____
2._____	2._____
3._____	3._____
4._____	4._____
5._____	5._____

Why are these women important to you? Is it their personalities? Their spirituality? Their inner strength? Is their body size an influential factor?

If you found it difficult to identify important women in your life, explore the reasons why. Some women have said to me, "I'm too fat to have close female friendships. When I lose weight, I'll seek out my support system in the female community." This comment is yet another example of how we put our lives on hold until we lose weight. Dieting and the quest for thinness have isolated women, separated the female community, and caused competitiveness. When we walk into a room, we scan the bodies of other women for the "thinnest of them all." Then we are secretly jealous of those women who have a "better" body than we do—and we are secretly rejoicing when one of them gains weight.

The quest for a new relationship with food can bring us together! Seek out the help, support, nurturance, and guidance you need from your own female community—and model for your daughter the importance of female relationships. Then help others as you were helped. As a friend, how can you assist other women in developing a healthy relationship with food? How can you assist your friend's daughters? As an aunt, how can you help your niece? As a woman, how can you help your female community and contribute to the current and future generations of women? Keep in mind that one of the most important ways you can help others is to help yourself by changing your own relationship with food and your body—and by modeling a diet-free lifestyle.

By receiving social support *and* giving social support, you will initiate social change. Women comprise 52 percent of the population—we are the majority! By working together, we can establish a healthy eating legacy and ensure its passage to future generations of women.

THE HEALTHY EATING FUTURE—A REALITY TODAY

We have dieting to thank for our rediscovered joy with food. As soon as I, my mother, and my daughter gave up dieting, everything started falling into place. But how will I know when we've fully established healthier food relationships?

—Rose, age 37

Many mothers have asked me the same question Rose did: "How will I know when we have achieved healthier food and body relationships?" You'll be aware of so many changes and benefits that you can't help but know. You'll wake up one day realizing that:

- It's January 1 and you have no need to think about making a New Year's resolution to lose the weight you gained over the holidays—because you didn't gain any.

- It's Halloween, and your daughter is as excited about her costume as the candy.

- It's Valentine's Day, and your mother eats a couple of pieces of chocolate instead of devouring her usual pound within an hour.

- It's lunchtime, and your daughter is hungrier than usual because she's in a growth spurt, and you don't even think about questioning her food needs.

- It's Saturday afternoon, you open the cupboard for a snack, and your six-year-old daughter asks you, "What are you hungry for, Mom?"

- You just got off the phone with your mother, and it dawns on you that she didn't ask a single question about your weight.

As you are moving toward this wonderful day, the following questionnaire will give you the confirmation that you are headed in the right direction. The questions are worded to reflect the process more than the end result. For example, with the first question, "Are you respecting your body?" if you are respecting it more than you did before reading this book, then your answer is "yes." I purposefully did not phrase the question "Do you respect your body?" because you may answer "No, I do not respect my body yet" instead of "Yes, I am respecting my body more"—which indicates that change is in process.

Are You Establishing Healthier Food and Body Relationships?

	YOU	YOUR DAUGHTER	YOUR MOTHER
1. Are you respecting your body?	_____	_____	_____
2. Are you accepting the healthy biological passage of womanhood?	_____	_____	_____
3. Are you eating when you are hungry?	_____	_____	_____
4. Are you eating what you are hungry for?	_____	_____	_____
5. Are you eating the amount to satisfy your hunger?	_____	_____	_____
6. Are you eating your favorite foods?	_____	_____	_____
7. Are you eating a variety of foods?	_____	_____	_____
8. Are you satisfying your food cravings?	_____	_____	_____
9. Are your eating habits changing daily?	_____	_____	_____
10. Are you eating what you want in public?	_____	_____	_____
TOTAL NUMBER OF "YES" ANSWERS	_____	_____	_____

The greater the number of "yes" answers, the closer you, your daughter, and your mother are to achieving your personal transformation to instinctive eating.

When you are ready, you can also go back to pages 91 and 113 to retake the questionnaires "Do You Need to Work as a Team to Build Body Image and Self-Esteem?" and "Do You Need Some Latitude in Your Food Attitude?" Measuring changes can be validating *and* motivating.

With all the questionnaires in this book, none demands a perfect score. There is also no such thing as a perfect instinctive eater because the range of healthy, acceptable eating behaviors is too wide and imprecise to be perfect. Occasional overeating is a part of instinctive eating. Sometimes eating chocolate just for the sake of eating chocolate is a part of instinctive eating. Deciding to eat caviar just because you're at a party is a part of instinctive eating. And *not* feeling guilty about these behaviors is a part of instinctive eating.

With your heightened awareness of how disordered eating passes from generation to generation, of what is needed to change

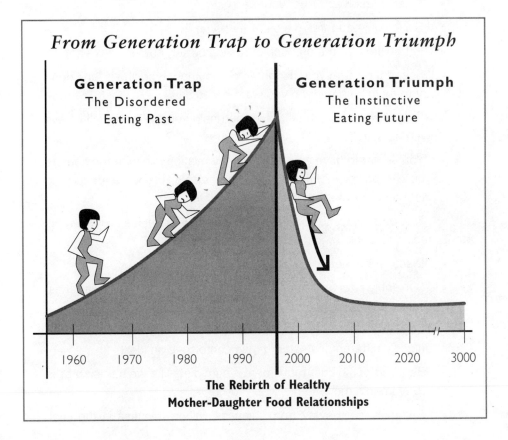

From Generation Trap to Generation Triumph

Generation Trap
The Disordered
Eating Past

Generation Triumph
The Instinctive
Eating Future

1960   1970   1980   1990   2000   2010   2020   3000

**The Rebirth of Healthy
Mother-Daughter Food Relationships**

189

to way you relate to food and your body, and of how to establish healthier mother-daughter food relationships, *you will achieve the instinctive eating future.*

As we look forward to the instinctive eating future and enter the twenty-first century, what advice would you give to the next generation of mothers? This was the final question asked to my focus groups and the closing question posed to the hundreds of women I interviewed. Without knowing the contents or philosophy of this book, here is just a sampling of their answers:

- "Don't be concerned about your daughter's eating habits, be concerned about yours—because yours will become hers."
- "Eat when you're hungry, let your daughter eat when she's hungry, and don't stress out about it."
- "Trust yourself and trust your daughter."
- "Raise your daughter in a diet-free home."
- "Eat healthy for the purpose of feeling better, not losing weight."
- "Spend time with your daughter, get to know who she is, and don't try to mold her into who you want her to be."
- "Fall in love with yourself, and then help your daughter fall in love with herself."
- "You've got to have your own healthy relationship with food before you can positively influence anybody else's. If you won't give up dieting for yourself, do it for your daughter."
- "Find other ways to nurture your children, whether it's taking a walk, reading a book, or just listening to them."
- "Discover hunger."
- "Put energy toward important issues instead of superficial ones. Dieting is superficial, nourishment is important."
- "Celebrate what's wonderful about each of you, focus on what's uniquely different instead of trying conform to an ideal."
- "Be a part of a bigger movement—burn diets like we burned bras in the women's movement."
- "Redefine goals away from thinness. When thinness is the goal,

weight and food are the enemies. But when comfort in one's body is the goal, then weight and food are allies, and dieting and thinness are the enemies."

- "Chocolate is just fine, bread is just fine, cheese is just fine, meat is just fine—everything is just fine."
- "Put media influences in perspective."
- "Indulge in your favorite foods, learn to love your thighs, and celebrate being women over a meal together."

As you can see, these mothers predicted much of the advice given in this book. Instinctively, they knew *what* needed to be done to ensure a healthy eating legacy. Before reading this book, you instinctively knew too; I've simply outlined *how* to do it and *why* we need to do it—*now.*

My personal and professional experience has taught me that the journey to healthier food and body relationships begins by giving up dieting, is propelled by education and an appreciation of the female body, and ends with the many rewards of body acceptance and eating enjoyment. I hope that I have imparted this knowledge and successfully guided you and the other important women in your life in your journeys.

You may have been unknowingly passing on the legacy of disordered eating, but now you have the wisdom and skills to knowingly pass on the legacy of instinctive eating to your daughter, granddaughter, and all future generations of women. Being a mother is the most challenging and rewarding experience of your life—and the same is true of being a daughter. Rise to the challenge and embrace the rewards. Together, your kinship, love, and instinct will lead the way.

Mothers, Daughters, and Food: A Summary of Findings from Focus Group Interviews

Laura E. Nathan, PhD, and Christine Lafia, PhD

The findings from four focus group interviews revealed that food is often a potent force in interpersonal relationships, especially the mother-daughter relationship. When focus group participants reflected on their mothers' influence on their feelings about food and their bodies, they cited both positive and negative influences. A few noted that their mothers served as healthy role models for eating habits and body acceptance. Others noted that food was linked to sociability or that, in their childhood, it was equated to comfort or love. The majority, however, recalled constant criticism of their bodies and/or what they were eating. The daughters interpreted this criticism to indicate a lack of acceptance—not just of their bodies or their food choices, but of themselves as persons.

Specifically, participants remembered their mothers monitoring how much they ate and sending direct or indirect messages to limit food consumption. Most focus group participants who were exposed to these messages during childhood had mothers who emphasized appearance. These daughters came to "know" that being overweight was unacceptable; in fact, several came to believe that being overweight meant being unhappy. These beliefs persisted into adulthood, with the daughters continuing to limit their own food consumption.

For most participants, food restriction through dieting began when they were girls or early teenagers, and many reported repeated cycles of weight loss and gain throughout their lives. Some stated that they had dieted with family members—sometimes sisters, but most often mothers. Several felt their dieting behaviors were related to the fact that their mothers were vigilant for any sign of weight gain. One woman reported that her mother consulted a diet doctor for her as soon as she reached puberty. After being placed on amphetamines at age fifteen, she blacked out. The message that these women received from their mothers while growing up became ingrained: to be female meant to struggle with one's weight, and that meant dieting.

Mothers, however, are not the only ones who influence women's feelings about or use of food. Nor are mothers the only ones who have an impact on how daughters feel about their bodies. Many of the focus group participants reported that important men in their lives, specifically fathers and husbands, have affected their ideas about eating and their bodies. Some recollected instances where their husbands exerted pressure on them, typically through requests or demands to lose weight. Others recalled their fathers giving them messages about the acceptability or unacceptability of their bodies.

Virtually all focus group participants felt their parents' attitudes and behaviors were linked to larger social forces at work in our culture. They spoke about the notion of the "ideal" woman prevalent in our society, based on appearance; this ideal is reinforced in the mass media and tells women that in order to be attractive, they need to be skinny. This desire to be unnaturally thin sets up a dynamic that can easily lead to an unhealthy relationship with food. Women are thus encouraged to become dependent on their mirrors and scales for a sense of self. As a consequence of these cultural messages and subsequent attempts to achieve the ideal, real women become unhappy with who they are. Their appearance can never live up to the ideal.

What advice would these focus group participants give to the next generation of mothers in order to encourage them to raise daughters who have healthy relationships with food? What do they believe constitutes a healthy mother-daughter food relationship? Most respondents advised mothers of the future to:

- Be aware of their own eating habits and patterns, so that they could set good examples for their daughters.
- Emphasize that food is to be enjoyed and make this clear by enjoying food with their daughters.
- Help daughters be happy with everything about themselves—including their bodies.

Perhaps more than anything else, these women believe that it is important to **minimize food as an issue**—to deemphasize it, so that it will not become a focal point in the lives of the next generation of women. Along these lines, participants recommended that future mothers encourage their daughters to:

- Eat what they like.
- Eat when they are hungry (and not at other times).
- Listen to their bodies.

One final note. The focus group method is powerful because it gives participants the opportunity to express their views as they interact with others on a specific topic. During these interviews, ideas develop as individuals discuss their thoughts in a group setting, and each member has the opportunity to have her voice heard. Every woman who participated in a focus group interview for this study had preidentified herself as having had an issue with food and what she would consider disordered eating. Virtually all the participants already had sought counsel for their eating problems—some through workshops and some through individual consultation. Since the participants were all volunteers who had identified themselves as having had disordered eating, it is important to be cautious when attempting to generalize about women and their relationships to food based solely on findings from these groups. However, considering the influence of society and a culture that focuses on food and objectifies women's bodies, the findings discussed here are likely suggestive of widespread patterns.

INTRODUCTION

1. S. C. Wooley et al., "Feeling Fat in a Thin Society," *Glamour Magazine* (February 1984):198.
2. L. M. Mellin et al., "Prevalence of Disordered Eating in Girls: A Survey of Middle Class Children," *Journal of the American Dietetic Association* 92(1992):851.
3. Wooley et al., "Feeling Fat in a Thin Society."
4. D. Greenfield et al., "Eating Behavior in an Adolescent Population," *International Journal of Eating Disorders* 6(1987):99.
5. Wooley et al., "Feeling Fat in a Thin Society."

CHAPTER ONE

1. J. Dwyer et al., "Potential Dieters: Who Are They?" *Journal of the American Dietetic Association* 56(1970):510; M. G. Stephenson et al., "The 1985 NHIS Findings: Nutrition Knowledge and Baseline Data for the Weight Loss Objectives," *Public Health Reports* 102(1987):61.
2. J. J. Sternlieb et al., "A Survey of Health Problems, Practices, and Needs of Youth," *Pediatrics* 49(1972):177; L. M. Mellin et al., "Prevalence of Disordered Eating in Girls: A Survey of Middle Class Children," *Journal of the American Dietetic Association,* 92(1992):851.
3. Mellin et al., "Prevalence of Disordered Eating in Girls."
4. S. C. Wooley et al., "Feeling Fat in a Thin Society," *Glamour Magazine* (February 1984):198.
5. A. Miller et al., "Diets Incorporated," *Newsweek,* September 11, 1989, 56.
6. M. T. Maloney et al., "Dieting Behavior and Eating Attitudes in Children," *Pediatrics* 84(1989):482.
7. W. Feldman et al., "Culture versus Biology: Children's Attitudes Towards Thinness and Fatness," *Pediatrics* 81(1988):190.
8. M. E. Collins, "Body Figure Perceptions and Preferences among Preadolescent Children," *International Journal of Eating Disorders* 10(1991):199.
9. Mellin et al., "Prevalence of Disordered Eating in Girls."
10. Ibid.
11. R. C. Hawkins et al., "Desirable and Undesirable Masculine and Feminine Traits in Relation to Students' Dietary Tendencies and Body Image Satisfaction," *Sex Roles* 9(1983):705.
12. M. Story et al., "Demographic and Risk Factors Associated with Chronic Dieting in Adolescents," *American Journal of Diseases of Children* 145(1991):994.
13. D. Greenfield et al., "Eating Behavior in an Adolescent Population," *International Journal of Eating Disorders,* 6(1987):99.

14. W. Feldman et al., "Adolescents' Pursuit of Thinness," *American Journal of Diseases of Children* 140(1986):294.
15. M. Nidiffer et al., "Attributes and Perceived Body Image of Students Seeking Nutrition Counseling in a University Wellness Program," *Journal of the American Dietetic Association,* Supplement 92(1992):A-56.
16. American School Public Health Association, Society for Public Health Education, *The National Adolescent Health Survey: A Report on the Health of America's Youth* (Oakland, Calif.: Third Party Publishing, 1989).
17. D. Neumark-Sztainer et al., "Dieting and Binge Eating: Which Dieters Are at Risk?" *Journal of the American Dietetic Association* 95(1995): 586.
18. R. J. Kuczmarski et al., "Increasing Prevalence of Overweight among US Adults," *Journal of the American Medical Association* 272(1994):205.
19. S. L. Gortmaker et al., "Increasing Pediatric Obesity in the United States," *American Journal of Diseases of Children* 141(1987):535.

CHAPTER 2

1. E. Koff et al., "Perceptions of Weight and Attitudes Toward Eating in Early Adolescent Girls," *Journal of Adolescent Health,* 12(1991):307.
2. K. T. Bundy, "Nutritional Adequacy of Snacks and Sources of Total Sugar Intake among US Adolescents," *Journal of the Canadian Dietetic Association* 43(1982):358.
3. L. L. Birch et al., "Eating as the 'Means' Activity in a Contingency: Effects on Young Children's Food Preferences," *Child Development* 51(1984):856.
4. P. R. Costanzo et al., "Domain-specific Parenting Styles and Their Impact on the Child's Development of Particular Deviance: The Example of Obesity Proneness," *Journal of Social and Clinical Psychology* 3(1985):425.
5. S. J. Foman, *Infant Nutrition,* 2nd ed. (Philadelphia: W. B. Saunders, 1974).
6. J. Morgan et al., "Factors Discriminating Restrained and Unrestrained Eaters: A Retrospective Self-report Study." Unpublished manuscript, 1985.
7. J. B. McCann et al., "The Eating Habits and Attitudes of Mothers of Children with Nonorganic Failure to Thrive," *Archives of Disease in Childhood* 70(1994):234.
8. S. Orbach, *Fat Is a Feminist Issue* (New York: Berkley Books, 1978), p. 18.
9. S. L. Johnson et al., "Parents' and Children's Adiposity and Eating Style," *Pediatrics* 94(1994):653.
10. Costanzo et al., "Domain-specific Parenting Styles and Their Impact on the Child's Development of Particular Deviance."
11. D. M. Garner et al., "Confronting the Failure of Behavioral and Dietary Treatment for Obesity," *Clinical Psychology Review* 11(1991):729.
12. K. M. Pike et al., "Mothers, Daughters, and Disordered Eating," *Journal of Abnormal Psychology* 100(1991):198.
13. R. J. Kuczmarski et al., "Increasing Prevalence of Overweight among US

Adults," *Journal of the American Medical Association* 272(1994):205.

14. A. T. Fleming, "Daughters of Dieters," *Glamour Magazine* (November 1994):222.

15. A. M. Gustafson-Larson et al., "Weight-related Behaviors and Concerns of Fourth Grade Children," *Journal of the American Dietetic Association* 92(1992):818.

16. B. M. Posner et al., "Secular Trends in Diet and Risk Factors of Cardiovascular Disease: The Framingham Study," *Journal of the American Dietetic Association* 95(1995):171; T. A. Nicklas, "Dietary Studies of Children: The Bogalusa Heart Study Experience," *Journal of the American Dietetic Association* 95(1995):1127.

17. C. Kies et al., "Family Pattern Similarities and Differences among Family Members," *Journal of the American Dietetic Association,* Supplement 92(1992):A-53.

18. Fleming, "Daughters of Dieters."

19. Ibid.

20. Pike et al., "Mothers, Daughters, and Disordered Eating."

21. S. C. Wooley et al, "Feeling Fat in a Thin Society," *Glamour Magazine* (February 1984):198.

22. M. Sigman-Grant, "Feeding Preschoolers: Balancing Nutritional and Developmental Needs," *Nutrition Today* (July/August 1992):13.

23. H. Canning et al., "Obesity: Its Possible Effect of College Acceptance," *New England Journal of Medicine* 275(1966):1172.

24. S. L. Gortmaker et al., "Social and Economic Consequences of Overweight in Adolescence and Young Adulthood," *New England Journal of Medicine* 329(1993):1008.

25. Ibid.

26. M. G. Efran, "The Effect of Physical Appearance, Interpersonal Attraction, and Severity of Recommended Punishment in a Simulated Jury Task," *Journal of Research in Personality* 8(1974):45.

27. M. Nasser, "Culture and Weight Consciousness," *Psychosomatic Research* 32(1988):573.

28. Ibid.

29. S. Rubin, "Why Samoans Can't Figure Out America's Diet Mania," *San Francisco Chronicle,* July 6, 1982, 17.

CHAPTER 3

1. G. C. Patton et al., "Abnormal Eating Attitudes in London Schoolgirls—a Prospective Epidemiological Study: Outcome at Twelve Month Follow-up," *Psychological Medicine* 20(1990):383.

2. Gallup Organization. "Women's Knowledge and Behavior Regarding Health and Fitness." Research conducted for the American Dietetic Association and Weight Watchers. June 1993.

3. J. H. Lacy et al., "Bulimia: Factors Associated with Its Etiology and Maintenance," *International Journal of Eating Disorders* 5(1986):472.

4. Patton et al., "Abnormal Eating Attitudes in London Schoolgirls."

5. R. R. Radcliffe, "What a New Study Reveals about Eating Disorders," *Shape Magazine* (October 1987):78.

6. M. Story et al., "Demographic and Risk Factors Associated with Chronic Dieting on Adolescents," *American Journal of Diseases of Children* 145(1991):994.
7. H. G. Pope et al., "Prevalence of Anorexia Nervosa and Bulimia in Three Student Populations," *International Journal of Eating Disorders* 3(1984):45.
8. American Psychiatric Association, *Diagnosis and Statistical Manual of Mental Disorders,* 4th ed. (Washington, D.C.: American Psychiatric Association, 1994), p. 544.
9. L. M. Mellin et al., "Prevalance of Disordered Eating in Girls: A Survey of Middle Class Children," *Journal of the American Dietetic Association* 92(1992):851.
10. W. Feldman, "Adolescents' Pursuit of Thinness," *American Journal of Diseases of Children.* 140(1986):294.
11. F. D. Kurtzman et al., "Eating Disorders among Select Female Student Populations at UCLA," *Journal of the American Dietetic Association* 89(1989):45.
12. J. Gray et al., "The Incidence of Bulimia in a College Sample," *International Journal of Eating Disorders* 4(1985):201.
13. "Newsbreaks: USDA Research Highlights," *Nutrition Today* 29(1994):5.
14. Mellin et al., "Prevalence of Disordered Eating in Girls."
15. "When Growing Pains Hurt Too Much: Teens at Risk," *Tufts University Diet and Nutrition Letter* 6(1991):3.
16. M. T. Pugliese et al., "Fear of Obesity: A Cause of Short Stature and Delayed Puberty," *New England Journal of Medicine* 309(1983):513.
17. L. Kaufman et al., "Children of the Corn," *Newsweek,* August 28, 1995, 60.
18. "Fat Free Foods: A Dieter's Downfall," *Environmental Nutrition* 18(1995):4.
19. "Periscope," *Newsweek,* August 28, 1995, 8.
20. D. J. Shide et al., "Information about the Fat Content of Preloads Influences Energy Intake in Healthy Women," *Journal of the American Dietetic Association* 95(1995):993.
21. D. C. Moore, "Body Image and Eating Behavior in Adolescent Girls," *American Journal of Diseases of Children* 142(1988):1114.
22. American Association of University Women, *AAUW Report: Short-changing Girls, Shortchanging America. Full Data Report* (Washington, DC: American Association of University Women, 1990), p. 19.
23. R. Freedman, *Bodylove* (New York: Perennial Library, 1988), 25.
24. M. Pipher, *Reviving Ophelia* (New York: Ballantine Books, 1994), 22.
25. W. Feldman et al., "Culture versus Biology: Children's Attitudes towards Thinness and Fatness," *Pediatrics* 81(1988):190.

CHAPTER 4

1. S. de Beauvoir as quoted in M. Pipher, *Reviving Ophelia* (New York: Ballantine Books, 1994), 57.

2. G. B. Slap et al., *Teenage Health Care* (New York: Pocket Books, 1994), 9.
3. M. P. Levine et al., "Normative Developmental Changes and Dieting and Eating Disturbances in Middle School Girls," *International Journal of Eating Disorders* 15(1994):11.
4. T. F. Cash et al., "The Great American Shape Up," *Psychology Today* (April 11, 1986):30.
5. "Obesity: New Directions in Treatment," *Nutrition and the MD* 21(1995):1.
6. D. E. Smith et al., "Longitudinal Changes in Adiposity Associated with Pregnancy," *Journal of the American Medical Association* 271(1994): 1747.
7. S. Potter et al., "Does Infant Feeding Method Influence Maternal Postpartum Weight Loss?" *Journal of the American Dietetic Association* 91(1991):441.
8. "Middle Age Spread," *Harvard Women's Health Watch* (August 1995):6.
9. K. G. Losonczy et al., "Does Weight Loss from Middle Age to Old Age Explain the Inverse Weight Mortality in Old Age?" *American Journal of Epidemiology* 141(1995):312.
10. W. C. Willett et al., "Weight, Weight Change, and Coronary Heart Disease in Women," *Journal of the American Medical Association* 273(1995):461; "Second Time Around: Weight Study Gets Pounded," *Women's Health Advocate Newsletter* 2(1995):6.
11. D. F. Williamson et al., "The 10 Year Incidence of Overweight and Major Weight Gain in US Adults," *Archives of Internal Medicine* 150(1990):665.
12. W. C. Knowler et al. "Diabetes Incidence in Pima Indians: Contribution of Obesity and Parental Diabetes," *American Journal of Epidemiology* 113(1981):144.
13. C. Bouchard, "Current Understanding of the Etiology of Obesity: Genetic and Nongenetic Factors," *American Journal of Clinical Nutrition* 55(1991):1561S.
14. S. L. Johnson et al., "Parents' and Children's Adiposity and Eating Style," *Pediatrics* 94(1994):653.
15. R. J. Kuczmarski et al., "Increasing Prevalence of Overweight among US Adults," *Journal of the American Medical Association* 272(1994):205.
16. S. Kumanyika et al., "Weight-related Attitudes and Behaviors of Black Women," *Journal of the American Dietetic Association* 93(1993):416.
17. S. M. Desmond et al., "Black and White Adolescent Perception of Their Weight," *Journal of School Health* 59(1989):353.
18. M. Ingrassia et al., "The Body of the Beholder," *Newsweek*, April 24, 1995, 66.
19. American Association of University Women, *AAUW Report: Shortchanging Girls, Shortchanging America. Full Data Report.* Washington, DC: American Association of University Women, 1990, p. 19.
20. M. Ingrassia et al., "The Body of the Beholder."
21. H. E. Marano et al., *Style Is Not a Size* (New York: Bantam Books, 1991), 23.

22. J. Stevens et al., "Attitudes Towards Body Size and Dieting: Differences between Elderly Black and White Women," *American Journal of Public Health* 84(1994):1322.

23. J. J. Gray et al., "The Prevalence of Bulimia in a Black College Population," *International Journal of Eating Disorders* 6(1987):733.

24. Kuczmarski et al., "Increasing Prevalence of Overweight among US Adults."

25. M. Story et al., "Weight Perceptions and Weight Control Practices in American Indian and Alaska Native Adolescents: A National Survey," *Archives of Pediatric and Adolescent Health* 148(1994):567.

26. M. Story et al., "Demographic and Risk Factors Associated with Chronic Dieting in Adolescence," *American Journal of Diseases of Children* 1(1991):994.

27. J. Wardle et al., "Culture and Body Image: Body Perception and Weight Concern in Young Asian and Caucasian British Women," *Journal of Community and Applied Social Psychology* 3(1993):173.

28. S. L. Anderson, "A Look at the Japanese Dietary Guidelines," *Journal of the American Dietetic Association* 90(1990):1527.

CHAPTER 5

1. P. Orenstein, *School Girls* (New York: Doubleday, 1994), xviii.

2. J. K. Thompson, "Larger than Life," *Psychology Today* (April 1986):38.

3. P. W. Moser, "Double Vision: Why Do We Never Match Up to Our Mind's Ideal?" *Self Magazine* (January 1989):51.

4. O. F. Lampley, "The Wig and I," *Mirabella* (March 1993):144.

5. "Vital Statistics," *Health Magazine* (March/April 1993):12.

6. D. C. Moore, "Body Image and Eating Behavior in Adolescent Girls," *American Journal of Diseases of Children* 142(1988):1114.

7. T. Watson et al., "Are You Too Fat?" *US News & World Report,* January 8, 1996, 52.

8. R. L. Leibel, et al., "Changes in Energy Expenditure Resulting from Altered Body Weight," *New England Journal of Medicine* 332(1995):621.

9. A. M. Gustafson-Larson et al., "Weight-related Behaviors and Concerns of Fourth-grade Children," *Journal of the American Dietetic Association* 92(1992):818.

10. L. Brody, "Are We Losing Our Girls?" *Shape Magazine* (November 1995):94.

CHAPTER 6

1. Gallup Organization, "Gallup Survey of Public Opinion Regarding Diet and Health." Prepared for the American Dietetic Association (Princeton, N.J.: Gallup Organization, 1990).

2. E. Koff et al., "Perception of Weight and Attitudes towards Eating in Early Adolescent Girls," *Journal of Adolescent Health* 12(1991):307.

3. L. Brody, "Fat Phobia," *Shape Magazine* (March 1993):104.

4. S. T. Borra et al., "Food, Physical Activity and Fun: Inspiring Ameri-

ca's Kids to More Healthful Lifestyles," *Journal of the American Dietetic Association* 95(1995):816.

5. Brody, "Fat Phobia."

6. Borra et al., "Food, Physical Activity and Fun."

7. J. Hastings, "Lip Service," *Health Magazine* (October 1992):73.

8. Koff et al., "Perception of Weight and Attitudes Towards Eating in Early Adolescent Girls."

9. "Diet Ads Sabotage Diets," *Tufts University Diet and Nutrition Letter* 13(1995):1.

10. "Chromium Picolinate Claims Thin on Evidence," *Tufts University Diet and Nutrition Letter* 13(1995):2.

11. L. Konner, "This Diet Pill's for Real," *Fitness* (September 1995):68.

12. E. Somer, "Crank It Up," *Shape Magazine* (October 1994):62.

13. "Smart Students, Foolish Choices," *Tufts University Diet and Nutrition Letter* 11(1993):2.

14. M. O'Neill, "So It May Be True After All: Eating Pasta Makes You Fat," *New York Times,* February 8, 1995, 1.

15. D. Webb, "Does Pasta Make You Fat?" *American Health* (October 1995):80.

16. L. Williams, "Stalking the Elusive Healthy Diet," *New York Times,* October 11, 1995, C1.

17. K. Napier, "Eggs," *American Health* (November 1995):75.

18. P. Long, "America's Top Food Myths," *Health* (October 1992):64.

19. M. Ternus, "Sugar and Kids: Not Necessarily a Dastardly Duo," *Environmental Nutrition* 14(1991):1.

20. J. J. Powell et al., "The Effects of Different Percentages of Dietary Fat Intake, Exercise, and Caloric Restriction on Body Composition and Body Weight in Obese Women," *American Journal of Health Promotion* 8(1994):442.

21. A. S. Murphy et al., "Kindergarten Students' Food Preferences Are Not Consistent with Their Knowledge of the Dietary Guidelines," *Journal of the American Dietetic Association* 95(1995):219.

22. Ibid.

CHAPTER 7

1. C. M. Davis, "Self-selection of Diet by Newly Weaned Infants: An Experimental Study," *American Journal of Diseases of Children* 36(1928):651.

2. L. L. Birch et al., "The Variability of Young Children's Energy Intake," *New England Journal of Medicine* 324(1991):232.

3. E. Koff et al., "Perceptions of Weight and Attitudes towards Eating in Early Adolescence," *Journal of Adolescent Health* 12(1991):307.

4. U.S. Bureau of the Census, *Statistical Abstract of the United States,* 110th ed. (Washington, DC: US Government Printing Office, 1991).

5. K. A. Rickard et al., "The Play Approach to Learning in the Context of Families and Schools: An Alternative Paradigm for Nutrition and Fitness Education in the 21st Century," *Journal of the American Dietetic Association* 95(1995):1121.

6. "Kids Are Surprisingly Nutrition Savvy," *Environmental Nutrition* (May 1992):3.
7. *Nutrition and Your Health: Dietary Guidelines for Americans,* 4th ed. U.S. Department of Agriculture. U.S. Department of Health and Human Services. Home and Garden Bulletin No. 232, 1995.
8. B. M. Posner et al., "Secular Trends in Diet and Risk Factors of Cardiovascular Disease: The Framingham Study," *Journal of the American Dietetic Association* 95(1995):171; T. A. Nicklas, "Dietary Studies of Children: The Bogalusa Heart Study Experience," *Journal of the American Dietetic Association* 95(1995):1127.
9. S. Cohen, "Have It Your Way," *Shape* (October 1995):82.
10. L. D. McBean, "Adolescent Nutrition: Issues and Challenges," *Dairy Council Digest* 58(1987):1.
11. "TV Food Ads Feed Kids the Wrong Messages," *Tufts University Diet and Nutrition Letter* 12(1995):7.
12. Ibid.
13. G. P. Sylvester et al., "Children's Television and Nutrition: Friends or Foes?" *Nutrition Today* 30(1995):6.
14. V. C. Strasberger, "Does Television Affect Learning and School Performance?" *Pediatrics* 13(1986):141.
15. "More on the Pitfalls of Television Watching," *Tufts University Diet and Nutrition Letter* 10(1992):6.
16. J. Martin, "Fitness Fun for the Whole Family," *American Health* (July/August 1995):70.
17. J. C. Singleton et al., "Role of Food and Nutrition in the Health Perceptions of Young Children," *Journal of the American Dietetic Association* 92(1992):68.
18. G. W. Heath et al., "Physical Activity Patterns in American High School Students: Results from the 1990 Youth Risk Behavior Study," *Archives of Pediatric and Adolescent Medicine* 148(1994):1131.
19. T. F. Cash et al., "The Great American Shape-up," *Psychology Today* (April 1986):30.
20. O. T. Raitakari et al., "Effects of Persistent Physical Activity on Coronary Risk Factors in Children and Young Adults," *American Journal of Epidemiology* 140(1994):195.
21. Martin, "Fitness Fun for the Whole Family."
22. S. Stallings et al., "Normal Weight Women," *Shape Magazine* (January 1990):34.
23. M. Wood, "Weight Loss: A Sex-linked Trait," *Agricultural Research* (August 1995):14.
24. Martin, "Fitness Fun for the Whole Family."
25. J. Polivy et al., "Undieting: A Program to Help People Stop Dieting," *International Journal of Eating Disorders* 11(1992):261.
26. P. Roughan et al., "Long-term Effects of a Physiologically Based Group Programme for Women Preoccupied with Weight and Eating Behavior," *International Journal of Obesity* 14(1990):135.
27. S. T. Borra et al., "Food, Physical Activity, and Fun: Inspiring America's Kids to More Healthy Lifestyles," *Journal of the American Dietetic Association* 95(1995):816.

28. F. E. M. Braddon et al., "Onset of Obesity in a 36-year Birth Cohort," *British Medical Journal* 293(1986):299.
29. L. R. Shapiro et al., "Obesity Prognosis: A Longitudinal Study of Children from the Age of 6 Months to 9 Years," *American Journal of Public Health* 74(1984):968.

CHAPTER 8

1. J. R. Rabinor, "Mother, Daughters and Eating Disorders: Honoring the Mother-Daughter Relationship." In P. Fallon, M. A. Katzman, and S. C. Wooley, *Feminist Perspectives on Eating Disorders* (New York: Guilford Press, 1994), 276.
2. "Mother's Day Marathon," *Shape Magazine* (May 1995):129.
3. A. Rich, *Of Women Born* (New York: W. W. Norton, 1986), 235.
4. M. K. Serdula et al., "Fruit and Vegetable Intake among Adults in 16 States: Results of a Brief Telephone Survey," *American Journal of Public Health* 85(1995):236.
5. R. R. Wing et al., "Effect of Modest Weight Loss on Changes in Cardiovascular Risk Factors: Are There Differences between Men and Women or between Weight Loss and Maintenance?" *International Journal of Obesity* 19(1995):67.
6. H. H. Keller, "Weight Gain Impacts Morbidity and Mortality in Institutionalized Older Persons," *Journal of the American Geriatrics Society* 43(1995):165.
7. "Newsbreaks: USDA Research Highlights," *Nutrition Today* 29(1994):4.
8. D. F. Williamson et al., "Weight Loss Attempts in Adults: Goals, Duration, and Rate of Weight Loss," *American Journal of Public Health* 82(1992):1251.
9. D. Goleman, "Eating Disorder Rates Surprise the Experts," *New York Times,* October 4, 1995, C11.
10. A. Drewnowski et al., "Men and Body Image: Are Men Satisfied with Their Body Weight?" *Psychsomatic Medicine* 49(1987):626.
11. A. Bierce, *The Devil's Dictionary* (New York: Dover, 1958). (Original work published 1911.)
12. American Association of University Women, *AAUW Report: Shortchanging Girls, Shortchanging America. Executive summary* (Washington, D.C.: American Association of University Women, 1991), 6.
13. R. C. Hawkins et al., "Desirable and Undesirable Masculine and Feminine Traits in Relation to Students, Dietary Tendencies and Body Image Satisfaction," *Sex Roles* 9(1983):705.
14. F. D. Kurtzman et al., "Eating Disorders among Select Female Student Population at UCLA," *Journal of the American Dietetic Association* 89(1989):45.
15. S. S. Fader, "Are Men Changing?" *Working Mother* (February 1993):49.
16. Ibid.

ADDITIONAL RESOURCES

WORKING AS A TEAM TO BUILD BODY IMAGE AND SELF-ESTEEM: A WORKBOOK TO HELP YOUNG WOMEN FEED AND RESPECT THE BODIES THEY WERE BORN WITH

Filled with activity sheets, assessments, thought-provoking questions, and journal pages for record keeping, this interactive workbook by Debra Waterhouse is designed to help the important 8- to 18-year-old in your life implement the many suggestions and activities shared in *Like Mother, Like Daughter*. To order, please send $10.00 plus $2.00 shipping and handling to:

Working As A Team
P.O. Box 4735,
Portland, ME 04112.

SEMINARS AND WORKSHOPS

If your organization is interested in a presentation on *Like Mother, Like Daughter* or any other women's health topic, please contact:

Debra Waterhouse
6114 LaSalle Avenue #342,
Oakland, CA 94611.

SHARING YOUR EXPERIENCES

If you would like to share your personal experiences in establishing healthier mother-daughter food relationships, please send letters to the above address.

SUGGESTED READING

Bingham, M., Edmondson, J., and Stryker S. *Choices: A Teen Woman's Journal for Self-awareness and Personal Planning*. Santa Barbara, Calif.: Advocacy Press, 1993.

Boston Women's Health Collective. *The New Our Bodies, Ourselves*. New York: Touchstone Books, 1992.

Brazelton, T. *Touchpoints*. New York: Addison Wesley, 1992.

Brumburg, J. J. *Fasting Girls*. Cambridge, Mass.: Harvard University Press, 1988.

Byrne, K. *A Parent's Guide to Anorexia and Bulimia*. New York: An Owl Book, 1987.

Caplan, P. J. *Don't Blame Mother*. New York: Perennial, 1989.

Chernin, K. *The Hungry Self*. New York: Times Books, 1985.

Debold, E., Wilson, M., and Malave, I. *Mother Daughter Revolution*. New York: Bantam Books, 1993.

Edelman, H. *Motherless Daughters*. New York: Delta Books, 1994.

Elium, J., and Elium, D. *Raising a Daughter*. Berkeley, Calif.: Celestial Arts, 1994.

Fallon, P., Katzman, M. A., and Wooley, S. C. *Feminist Perspectives on Eating Disorders*. New York: Guilford Press, 1994.

Foreyt, J. P., and Goodrick, G. K. *Living Without Dieting*. New York: Warner Books, 1992.

Freedman, R. *Bodylove*. New York: Perennial Library, 1988.

Goodman, L. J. *Is Your Child Dying to Be Thin?* Pittsburgh: Dorrance Publishing, 1992.

Hall, L. *Full Lives: Women Who Have Freed Themselves from Weight Obsessions*. Carlsbad, Calif.: Gurze Books, 1993.

Hall, L., and Cohn, L. *Self-Esteem: Tools for Recovery*. Carlsbad, Calif.: Gurze Books, 1990.

Hancock, E. *The Girl Within*. New York: Fawcett Columbine, 1989.

Hirschmann, J. R., and Munter, C. H. *Overcoming Overeating*. New York: Fawcett Columbine, 1988. (See "Organizations.")

Hirschmann, J. R., and Munter, C. H. *When Women Stop Hating Their Bodies*. New York: Fawcett Columbine, 1995.

Hirschmann, J. R., and Zaphiropoulos, L. *Preventing Childhood Eating Problems*. Carlsbad, Calif.: Gurze Books, 1993.

Hollis, J. *Fat Is a Family Affair*. San Francisco: Harper/Hazelden, 1985.

Hutchinson, M. G. *Transforming Body Image*. Freedom, Calif.: The Crossing Press, 1985.

Jackson, D. *How to Make the World a Better Place for Women in Five Minutes a Day*. New York: Hyperion, 1992.

Johnson, C. A. *Self-Esteem Comes in All Sizes*. New York: Doubleday, 1995.

Johnson, K. *Trusting Ourselves*. New York: The Atlantic Monthy Press, 1991.

Kano, S. *Making Peace with Food.* New York: Perennial Library, 1989.

Kleinman, R. E., Jellinek, M. S., and Houston, J. *What Should I Feed My Kids?* New York: Fawcett Columbine, 1994.

Kubersky, R. *Everything You Need to Know About Eating Disorders.* New York: Rosen Publishing Group, 1996.

Lansky, V. *Fat-Proofing Your Children.* New York: Bantam Books, 1988.

Levine. M. *How Schools Can Help Combat Student Eating Disorders.* National Education Association, Washington, D.C.: NEA Professional Library, 1987.

Maine, M. *Father Hunger: Fathers, Daughters, and Food.* Carlsbad, Calif.: Gurze Books, 1991.

Marano, H. E. *Style Is Not a Size.* New York: Bantam Books, 1991.

Mellin, L. *The Shapedown Solution: The Six True Cures of Weight Problems.* New York: The Regan Company, 1997.

———. *The Shapedown Weight Management Program for Children and Teens,* 5th ed. San Anselmo, Calif.: Balboa Publishing. 1992. (See "Organizations.")

Millman, M. *Such a Pretty Face.* New York: Berkley Books, 1980.

Northrup, C. *Women's Bodies, Women's Wisdom.* New York: Bantam Books, 1994.

Orbach, S. *Fat Is a Feminist Issue.* New York: Berkley Books, 1978.

———. *Fat Is a Feminist Issue II.* New York: Berkley Books, 1982.

———. *Hunger Strike.* New York: Avon Books, 1986.

Orenstein, P. *School Girls.* New York: Doubleday, 1994.

Pipher, M. *Reviving Ophelia.* New York: Ballantine Books, 1994.

Rodin, J. *Body Traps.* New York: Quill, 1992.

Roth, G. *Breaking Free from Compulsive Overeating.* New York: Bobbs-Merrill, 1990.

———. *Feeding the Hungry Heart.* New York: Bobbs-Merrill, 1982.

———. *When Food Is Love.* New York: Plume Books, 1991.

———. *Appetites.* New York: Dutton, 1996.

Satter, E. *How to Get Your Kid to Eat . . . But Not Too Much.* Palo Alto, Calif.: Bull Publishing, 1987.

Schroeder, C. R. *Fat Is Not a Four Letter Word.* Minneapolis: Chronimed, 1992.

Secunda, V. *When You and Your Mother Can't Be Friends.* New York: Delta Books, 1990.

———. *Women and Their Fathers.* New York: Delta Books, 1992.

Sied, R. P. *Never Too Thin: Why Women Are at War with Their Bodies.* New York: Prentice-Hall, 1989.

Siegel, M., Brisman, J., and Weinshel, M. *Surviving an Eating Disorder.* New York: Perennial, 1988.

Slap, G. B., and Jablow, M. M. *Teenage Health Care.* New York: Pocket Books, 1994.

Somer, E. *Nutrition for Women.* New York: Henry Holt and Co., 1993.

Stacey, M. *Consumed: Why Americans Love, Hate, and Fear Food.* New York: Simon and Schuster. 1994.

Tribole, E., and Resch, E. *Intuitive Eating.* New York: St. Martin's Press, 1995.

Waterhouse, D. *Outsmarting the Female Fat Cell.* New York: Warner Books, 1993.

——. *Why Women Need Chocolate.* New York: Hyperion, 1995.

Wexler, D. B. *The Adolescent Self.* New York: W. W. Norton, 1991.

Wolf, N. *The Beauty Myth.* New York: Anchor Books, 1991.

Zerbe, K. J. *The Body Betrayed.* Carlsbad, Calif.: Gurze Books, 1993.

American Dietetic Association
216 West Jackson Boulevard
Chicago, IL 60606
(800) 366-1655

Anorexia Nervosa and Related Eating Disorders Inc. (ANRED)
PO Box 5102
Eugene, OR 97405
(503) 344-1144

Largely Positive
PO Box 17223
Glendale, WI 52317

National Association of Anorexia Nervosa and Associated Disorders
(ANAD)
Box 7
Highland Park, IL 60035
(847) 831-3438

National Association to Advance Fat Acceptance (NAAFA)
PO Box 188620
Sacramento, CA 95818
(800) 442-1214

The National Center for Overcoming Overeating
PO Box 1257
Old Chelsea Station
New York, New York 10113
(212) 875-0442

National Eating Disorders Organization (NEDO)
445 E. Grandville Road
Worthington, OH 43085
(918) 481-4044

Shapedown Weight Management Program for Children and Teens
For locations nearest to your area, contact:

Balboa Publishing
11 Library Place
San Anselmo, CA 94960
(415) 453-8886; fax (415) 453-8888

Weight Control Information Network
National Institutes of Health
(800) WIN-8098

Women Insisting on Natural Shapes (WINS)
PO Box 19938
Sacramento, CA 95819
(800) 600-9467

Adame, D. D. "Physical Fitness in Relation to the Amount of Physical Exercise, Body Image, and Locus of Control among College Men and Women." *Perpetual and Motor Skills* 70(1990):1347.

Adams, L. B. et al. "Early Manifestations of Eating Disorders in Adolescents: Defining Those at Risk." *Journal of Nutrition Education* 20(1988):307.

American Association of University Women. *AAUW Report: Shortchanging Girls, Shortchanging America. Full Data Report.* Washington, DC: American Association of University Women, 1990.

American Association of University Women. *AAUW Report: Shortchanging Girls, Shortchanging America. Executive Summary.* Washington, DC: American Association of University Women, 1991.

American Psychiatric Association. *Diagnostic and Statistical Manual of Mental Disorders,* 4th ed. Washington, DC: American Psychiatric Association, 1994.

Anderson, J. J. B. "Dietary Calcium and Bone Mass through the Lifecycle." *Nutrition Today* (March/April 1990):9.

Anderson, S. L. "A Look at the Japanese Dietary Guidelines." *Journal of the American Dietetic Association* 90(1990):1527.

Attie, I. et al. "Development of Eating Problems in Adolescent Girls: A Longitudinal Study." *Developmental Psychology* 25(1989):70.

Barish, E. B. "Dieting May Be a Losing Proposition." *Harvard Health Letter* (August 1994):4.

Barr, S. I. et al. "Restrained Eating and Ovulatory Disturbances: Possible Implications for Bone Health." *American Journal of Clinical Nutrition* 59(1994):92.

Beatie, H. J. "Eating Disorders and the Mother-Daughter Relationship." *International Journal of Eating Disorders* 7(1988):453.

Bell, C. et al. "Body Image of Anorexic, Obese, and Normal Females." *Journal of Clinical Psychology* 42(1986):431.

Bierce, A. *The Devil's Dictionary.* New York: Dover. (Original work published 1911.)

Birch, L. L. et al. "Caloric Compensation and Sensory Specific Satiety. Evidence of Self-Regulation of Food Intake by Young Children." *Appetite* 7(1986): 323.

———. "Mother-Child Interaction Patterns and the Degree of Fatness in Children." *Journal of Nutrition Education* 13(1981):17.

———. "Eating as the 'Means' Activity in a Contingency: Effects on Young Children's Food Preferences." *Child Development* 51(1984):856.

———. "Conditioned and Unconditioned Caloric Compensation: Evidence of Self-Regulation of Food Intake by Young Children." *Learning and Motivation* 16(1985):341.

———. "The Variability of Young Children's Energy Intake." *New England Journal of Medicine* 324(1991):232.

Borra, S. T. et al. "Food, Physical Activity and Fun: Inspiring America's Kids to More Healthful Lifestyles." *Journal of the American Dietetic Association* 95(1995):816.

Bouchard, C. "Current Understanding of the Etiology of Obesity: Genetic and Nongenetic Factors." *American Journal of Clinical Nutrition* 55(1991): 1561S.

Bouchard, C. et al. "Inheritance of the Amount and Distribution of Human Body Fat." *International Journal of Obesity* 12(1988):205.

———. "The Response to Long-term Overfeeding in Identical Twins." *New England Journal of Medicine* 322(1990):1477.

Braddon, F. E. M. et al. "Onset of Obesity in a 36 Year Birth Cohort." *British Medical Journal* 293(1986):299.

Brazelton, T. B. *Touchpoints.* New York: Addison Wesley, 1992.

Brenner, J. B. et al. "Gender Differences in Eating Attitudes, Body Concept, and Self-esteem among Models." *Sex Roles* 27(1992):413.

Brinch, M. et al. "Anorexia Nervosa and Motherhood: Reproduction Pattern and Mothering Behavior of 50 Women." *Acta Psychiatrica Scaninavica* 77(1988):611.

Brody, L. "Fat Phobia." *Shape Magazine* (March 1993):104.

———. "Are We Losing Our Girls?" *Shape Magazine* (November 1995):94.

———. "Diets through the Decades." *Shape Magazine* (February 1996):96.

Brooks-Gunn, J. "Antecedents and Consequences of Variations in Girls' Maturational Timing." *Journal of Adolescent Health Care* 9(1988):1.

Brownwell, K. "Dieting and the Search for the Perfect Body: Where Physiology and Culture Collide." *Behavior Therapy* 22(1991):1.

Brownwell, K. D. et al. "The Dieting Maelstrom: Is It Possible and Advisable to Lose Weight?" *American Psychologist* 40(1994):781.

Bruce, B. et al. "Binge Eating in Females: A Population-based Investigation." *International Journal of Eating Disorders* 12(1992):365.

———. "Binge Eating among the Overweight Population: A Serious and Prevalent Problem." *Journal of the American Dietetic Association* 96(1996):58.

Bruch, H. *The Golden Cage.* Cambridge, Mass.: Harvard University Press, 1978.

Bull, N. L. "Studies of the Dietary Habits, Food Consumption and Nutrient Intakes of Adolescents and Young Adults." *World Review of Nutrition and Dietetics* 57(1988):24.

Bundy, K. T. "Nutritional Adequacy of Snacks and Sources of Total Sugar Intake among US Adolescents." *Journal of the Canadian Dietetic Association* 43(1982):358.

Calam, R. et al. "Eating Disorders and Perceived Relationships with Parents." *International Journal of Eating Disorders* 9(1990):479.

Canning, H. et al. "Obesity: Its Possible Effect on College Acceptance." *New England Journal of Medicine* 275(1966):1172.

Cash, T. F. et al. "The Great American Shape-up." *Psychology Today* (April 1986):30.

———. "Body Image in Anorexia Nervosa and Bulimia Nervosa." *Behavior Modification* 2(1987):487.

Casper, R. C. "Personality Features of Women with Good Outcome from Restricting Anorexia Nervosa." *Psychosomatic Medicine* 52(1990):156.

Cassel, J. "Social Anthropology and Nutrition: A Different Look at Obesity in America." *Journal of the American Dietetic Association* 95(1995):424.

Chan, G. M. et al. "Effects of Dairy Products on Bone and Body Composition in Pubertal Girls." *Journal of Pediatrics* 126(1995):551.

Charone, J. "Eating Disorders: Their Genesis in the Mother-Infant Relationship." *International Journal of Eating Disorders* 4(1982):15.

Chodorow, N. *The Reproduction of Mothering: Psychoanalysis and the Sociology of Gender*. Berkeley: University of California Press, 1978.

"Chromium Picolinate Claims Thin on Evidence." *Tufts University Diet and Nutrition Letter* 13(1995):2.

Cohen, S. "Have It Your Way." *Shape* (October 1995):82.

Collins, M. E. "Education for a Healthy Body Weight: Helping Adolescents Balance the Cultural Pressure for Thinness." *Journal of School Health* 58(1988):227.

———. "Body Figure Perceptions and Preferences among Preadolescent Children." *International Journal of Eating Disorders* 10(1991):199.

Conner-Greene, P. A. "Gender Differences in Body Weight Perception and Weight Loss Strategies of College Students." *Women and Health* 14(1988): 27.

Costanzo, P. R. et al. "Parental Perspectives on Obesity in Children: The Importance of Sex Differences." *Journal of Social and Clinical Psychology* 2(1984):305.

———. "Domain-specific Parenting Styles and Their Impact on the Child's Development of Particular Deviance: The Example of Obesity Proneness." *Journal of Social and Clinical Psychology* 3(1985):425.

Crisp, A. H. "Some Psychobiological Aspects of Adolescent Growth and Their Relevance for the Fat/Thin Syndrome." *International Journal of Obesity* 1(1977):231.

———. "Some Possible Approaches to Prevention of Eating and Body Weight/ Shape Disorders, with Particular Reference to Anorexia Nervosa." *International Journal of Eating Disorders* 7(1988):1.

Cross, A. T. et al. "Snacking Patterns among 1800 Adults and Children." *Journal of the American Dietetic Association* 94(1994):1398.

Cross, L. W. "Body and Self in Feminine Development: Implications for Eating Disorders and Delicate Self-mutilation." *Bulletin of the Menninger Clinic* 57(1993):41.

Czajka-Narins, D. M. et al. "Fear of Fat: Attitudes towards Obesity." *Nutrition Today* (January/February 1990):26.

Davis, C. M. "Self-selection of Diet by Newly Weaned Infants: An Experimental Study." *American Journal of Diseases of Children* 36(1928):651.

de Beauvoir, S. *The Second Sex*. New York: H. M. Parshley, 1971.

Desmond, S. M. et al. "Black and White Adolescent Perception of Their Weight." *Journal of School Health* 59(1989):353.

Devine, C. M. et al. "Women's Perception about the Way Social Roles Promote or Constrain Personal Nutrition Care." *Women and Health* 19(1992):79.

"Diet Ads Sabotage Diets." *Tufts University Diet and Nutrition Letter* 13(1995):1.

Dietz, W. H. "You Are What You Eat—What You Eat Is What You Are." *Journal of Adolescent Health Care* 11(1990):76.

———. "Critical Periods in Childhood for the Development of Obesity." *American Journal of Clinical Nutrition* 59(1994):955.

———. "Does Hunger Cause Obesity?" *Pediatrics* 95(1995):766.

Dietz, W. H. et al. "Do We Fatten Our Children at the Television Set? Obesity and Television Watching in Children and Adolescents." *Pediatrics* 75(1985): 807.

Drewnowski, A. et al. "Men and Body Image: Are Men Satisfied with Their Body Weight?" *Psychosomatic Medicine* 49(1987):626.

Drinkwater, B. L. et al. "Bone Mineral Content of Amenorrheic and Eumenorrheic Athletes." *New England Journal of Medicine* 311(1984):277.

Dugdale, A. E. et al. "The Effect of Lactation and Other Factors on Postpartum Changes in Body Weight and Triceps Skinfold Thickness." *British Journal of Nutrition* 61(1989):149.

Dwyer, J. et al. "Potential Dieters: Who Are They?" *Journal of the American Dietetic Association* 56(1970):510.

Edelman, H. *Motherless Daughters*. New York: Delta Books, 1994.

Efran, M. G. "The Effect of Physical Appearance, Interpersonal Attraction, and Severity of Recommended Punishment in a Simulated Jury Task." *Journal of Research in Personality* 8(1974):45.

Ehrensing, R. H. et al. "The Mother-Daughter Relationship in Anorexia Nervosa." *Psychosomatic Medicine* 32(1970):201.

Eiger, M. R. et al. "Change in Eating Attitudes: An Outcome Measure of Patients with Eating Disorders." *Journal of the American Dietetic Association* 96(1996):62.

Einstein, N. et al. "Prevalence of Eating Disorders among Dietetics Students: Does Nutrition Education Make a Difference?" *Journal of the American Dietetic Association* 92(1992):949.

Emmons, L. "Dieting and Purging Behavior in Black and White High School Students." *Journal of the American Dietetic Association* 92(1992):306.

———. "Predisposing Factors Differentiating Adolescent Dieters and Nondieters." *Journal of the American Dietetic Association* 94(1994):725.

Fader, S. S. "Are Men Changing?" *Working Mother* (February 1993):49.

Fallon, P., Katzman, M. A., and Wooley, S. C. *Feminist Perspectives on Eating Disorders*. New York: Guilford Press, 1994.

Faludi, S. *Backlash: The Undeclared War against American Women*. New York: Crown Books, 1991.

"Fat Free Foods: A Dieter's Downfall." *Environmental Nutrition* 18(1995):4.

Feldman, W. "Adolescents' Pursuit of Thinness." *American Journal of Diseases of Children* 140(1986):294.

Feldman, W. et al. "Culture versus Biology: Children's Attitudes towards Thinness and Fatness." *Pediatrics* 81(1988):190.

Fisher, J. O. et al. "Fat Preferences and Fat Consumption of 3- to 5-Year-Old Children Are Related to Parental Adiposity." *Journal of the American Dietetic Association* 95(1995):759.

Fleming, A. T. "Daughters of Dieters." *Glamour Magazine* (November 1994): 222.

Foltin, R. W. et al. "Caloric Compensation for Lunches Varying in Fat and Carbohydrate Content by Humans in a Residential Laboratory." *American Journal of Clinical Nutrition* 52(1990):969.

Foman, S. J. *Infant Nutrition,* 2nd ed. Philadelphia: W. B. Saunders, 1974.

Fontaine, K. L. "The Conspiracy of Culture: Women's Issues in Body Size." *Nursing Clinics of North America* 26(1991):669.

Forbes, G. B. "Children and Food: Order amid Chaos." *New England Journal of Medicine* 324(1991):262.

Foreyt, J. P. et al. "Weight Management without Dieting." *Nutrition Today* (March/April 1993):4.

Fornari, V. et al. "Anorexia Nervosa: 'Thirty something.' " *Journal of Substance Abuse Treatment* 11(1994):45.

Frank, G. C. et al. "A Food Frequency Questionnaire for Adolescents: Defining Eating Patterns." *Journal of the American Dietetic Association* 92(1992): 313.

Fredenberg, J. P. et al. "Incidence of Eating Disorders among Selected Female University Students." *Journal of the American Dietetic Association* 96(1996):64.

Freedman, R. *Bodylove.* New York: Perennial Library, 1988.

———. "Mind over Mirror." *Shape Magazine* (March 1991):98.

French, S. et al. "Food Preferences, Eating Patterns, and Physical Activity among Adolescents: Correlates of Eating Disorders Symptoms." *Journal of Adolescent Health* 15(1994):268.

Gallup Organization. "Gallup Survey of Public Opinion Regarding Diet and Health." Survey prepared for the American Dietetic Association. Princeton, N.J.: Gallup Organization, 1990.

———. "Women's Knowledge and Behavior Regarding Health and Fitness." Survey conducted for the American Dietetic Association and Weight Watchers, June 1990.

Garner, D. M. et al. "Cultural Expectations of Thinness in Women." *Psychology Reports* 47(1980):483.

———. "Socio-cultural Factors in the Development of Anorexia Nervosa." *Psychological Medicine* 10(1980):647.

———. "Comparison between Weight-preoccupied Women and Anorexia Nervosa." *Psychosomatic Medicine* 46(1984):255.

———. "Confronting the Failure of Behavioral and Dietary Treatment for Obesity." *Clinical Psychology Review* 11(1991):729.

Gilligan, C. *In a Different Voice.* Cambridge, Mass.: Harvard University Press, 1982.

Glassner, B. 1989. "Fitness and the Postmodern Self." *Journal of Health and Social Behavior* 30(1989):180.

Goldman, H. E. "Does She Deserve to Live? A Psychodynamic Case Study of an Anorexic Mother and Her Young Child." *International Journal of Eating Disorders* 7(1988):561.

Goleman, D. "Eating Disorder Rates Surprise the Experts." *New York Times,* October 4, 1995, C11.

Gortmaker, S. L. et al. "Inactivity, Diet, and the Fattening of America." *Journal of the American Dietetic Association* 90(1990):1247.

215

————. "Social and Economic Consequences of Overweight in Adolescence and Young Adulthood." *New England Journal of Medicine* 329(1993):1008.

Gray, J. et al. "The Incidence of Bulimia in a College Sample." *International Journal of Eating Disorders* 4(1985):201.

Gray, J. J. et al. "The Prevalence of Bulimia in a Black College Population." *International Journal of Eating Disorders* 6(1987):733.

Greenfield, D. et al. "Eating Behavior in an Adolescent Population." *International Journal of Eating Disorders* 6(1987):99.

Grunwald, K. L. "Weight Control in Young College Women." *Journal of the American Dietetic Association* 85(1985):1145.

Guillen, E. O. et al. "Nutrition, Dieting, and Fitness Messages in a Magazine for Adolescent Women, 1970–1990." *Journal of Adolescent Health* 15(1994):464.

Gustafson-Larson, A. M. et al. "Weight-related Behaviors and Concerns of Fourth-grade Children." *Journal of the American Dietetic Association* 92(1992):818.

Haines, P. A. et al. "Eating Patterns and Energy and Nutrient Intake of US Women." *Journal of the American Dietetic Association* 92(1992):698.

Halmi, K. A. et al. "Binge-eating and Vomiting: A Survey of a College Population." *Psychological Medicine* 11(1981):697.

Hampl, J. S. et al. "Comparisons of Dietary Intake and Sources of Fat in Low- and High-Fat Diets of 18- to 24-year-olds." *Journal of the American Dietetic Association* 95(1995):893.

Harding, T. P. et al. "Family Interaction Patterns and Locus of Control as Predictors of the Presence and Severity of Anorexia Nervosa." *Journal of Clinical Psychology* 42(1986):440.

Hastings, J. "Lip Service." *Health Magazine* (October 1992):73.

Hawkins, R. C. et al. "Desirable and Undesirable Masculine and Feminine Traits in Relation to Students' Dietary Tendencies and Body Image Satisfaction." *Sex Roles* 9(1983):705.

Heath, G. W. et al. "Physical Activity Patterns in American High School Students: Results from the 1990 Youth Risk Behavior Study." *Archives of Pediatric and Adolescent Medicine* 148(1994):1131.

Heilbraun, A. B. et al. "Distorted Body Image as a Risk Factor in Anorexia Nervosa: Replication and Clarification." *Psychological Reports* 66(1990):407.

Henderson, R. C. "Bone Health in Adolescence." *Nutrition Today* (March/April 1991):25.

Hill, A. J. "Dieting Concerns Have a Functional Effect on the Behavior of Nine-Year-Old Girls." *British Journal of Clinical Psychology* 30(1991):265.

Hill, A. J. et al. "Dieting Concerns of 10-Year-Old Girls and Their Mothers." *British Journal of Clinical Psychology* 29(1990):346.

————. "Eating in the Adult World: The Rise of Dieting in Childhood and Adolescence." *British Journal of Clinical Psychology* 31(1992):95.

Hoerr, S. L. et al. "Discrepancies among Predictors of Desirable Weight for Black and White Obese Adolescent Girls." *Journal of the American Dietetic Association* 92(1992):450.

Howat, P. M. et al. "The Influence of Diet, Body Fat, Menstrual Cycling, and

Activity upon the Bone Density of Females." *Journal of the American Dietetic Association* 89(1989):1305.

Hsu, L. K. et al. "Are Eating Disorders Becoming More Common in Blacks?" *International Journal of Eating Disorders* 6(1987):113.

Humphrey, L. L. "Family Relations in Bulimic-Anorexic and Nondistressed Families." *International Journal of Eating Disorders* 5(1986):223.

———. "Observed Family Interactions among Subtypes of Eating Disorders Using Structural Analysis of Social Behavior." *Journal of Consulting and Clinical Psychology* 57(1989):206.

Ingrassia, M. et al. "The Body of the Beholder." *Newsweek,* April 24, 1995, 66.

Jackson, E. G. "Family Meals More Important than Nutrition Perfection." *Environmental Nutrition* 13(1990):1.

Johnson, R. K. et al. "Effect of Maternal Employment on the Quality of Young Children's Diets: The CSFII Experience." *Journal of the American Dietetic Association* 92(1992):214.

Johnson, S. L. et al. "Conditioned Preferences: Young Children Prefer Flavors Associated with High Dietary Fat." *Physiological Behavior* 50(1991): 1245.

———. "Parents' and Children's Adiposity and Eating Style." *Pediatrics* 94(1994):653.

Jung, C. G. *The Collected Works of C. G. Jung: Vol. 9, Part 1. The Archetypes in the Collective Unconscious.* Princeton, N.J.: Princeton University Press, 1959.

Kaufman, L. et al. "Children of the Corn." *Newsweek,* August 28, 1995, 60.

Keller, H. H. "Weight Gain Impacts Morbidity and Mortality in Institutionalized Older Persons." *Journal of the American Geriatrics Society* 43(1995): 165.

Kelman, S. "Obsessed with Thin." *Shape Magazine,* July 1994, 76.

"Kids Are Surprisingly Nutrition Savvy." *Environmental Nutrition* (May 1992):3.

Kies, C. et al. "Family Pattern Similarities and Differences among Family Members." *Journal of the American Dietetic Association* (Supplement) 92(1992): A-53.

Killen, J. D. et al. "Self-induced Vomiting and Laxative and Diuretic Use among Teenagers: Precursors of the Binge-Purge Syndrome?" *Journal of the American Medical Association* 255(1986):1447.

———. "An Attempt to Modify Unhealthful Eating Attitudes and Weight Reduction Practices in Young Adolescent Girls." *International Journal of Obesity* 13(1993):369.

———. "Factors Associated with Eating Disorder Symptoms in a Community Sample of 6th and 7th Grade Girls." *International Journal of Eating Disorders* 15(1994):357.

King, G. A. et al. "Food Perceptions in Dieters and Nondieters." *Appetite* 8(1987):147.

Klesges, R. C. et al. "The Effects of Parental Influences on Children's Food Intake, Physical Activity, and Relative Weight." *International Journal of Eating Disorders* 5(1986):335.

———. "Parental Influence on Food Selection in Young Children and Its Relationship to Childhood Obesity." *American Journal of Clinical Nutrition* 53(1991):859.

———. "Effects of Television on Metabolic Rate: Potential Implications for Childhood Obesity." *Pediatrics* 91(1993):281.

———. "A Longitudinal Analysis of Accelerated Weight Gain in Preschool Children." *Pediatrics* 95(1995):126.

Knowler, W. C. et al. "Diabetes Incidence in Pima Indians: Contribution of Obesity and Parental Diabetes." *American Journal of Epidemiology* 113(1981):144.

Koff, E. et al. "Perception of Weight and Attitudes towards Eating in Early Adolescent Girls." *Journal of Adolescent Health* 12(1991):307.

Kog, E. et al. "Family Interaction in Eating Disorder Patients and Normal Controls." *International Journal of Eating Disorders* 8(1989):11.

Konner, L. "This Diet Pill's for Real." *Fitness* (September 1995):68.

Kramer F. M. et al. "Long-term Follow-up of Behavioral Treatment of Obesity: Patterns of Regain among Men and Women." *International Journal of Obesity* 13(1989):123.

Kreipe, R. E. et al. "Osteoporosis: A 'New Morbidity' for Dieting Female Adolescents?" *Pediatrics* 86(1990):478.

Kuczmarski, R. J. et al. "Increasing Prevalence of Overweight among US Adults." *Journal of the American Medical Association* 272(1994): 205.

Kumanyika, S. et al. "Weight-related Attitudes and Behaviors of Black Women." *Journal of the American Dietetic Association* 93(1993):416.

Kuntz, B., et al. "Bulimia: A Systemic Family History Perspective." *Families in Society* (December 1992):604.

Kurtzman, F. D. et al. "Eating Disorders among Select Female Student Population at UCLA." *Journal of the American Dietetic Association* 89(1989): 45.

Lacy, J. H. et al. "Bulimia: Factors Associated with Its Etiology and Maintenance." *International Journal of Eating Disorders* 5(1986):472.

Lampley, O. F. "The Wig and I." *Mirabella* (March 1993):144.

Leibel, R. L. et al. "Changes in Energy Expenditure Resulting from Altered Body Weight." *New England Journal of Medicine* 332(1995):621.

Levine, M. P. et al. "Normative Developmental Changes and Dieting and Eating Disturbances in Middle School Girls." *International Journal of Eating Disorders* 15(1994):11.

Lifshitz, F. et al. "Nutritional Dwarfing: Growth, Dieting, and Fear of Obesity." *Journal of the American College of Nutrition* 7(1988):367.

Lissner, L. et al. "Variability of Body Weight and Health Outcomes in the Framingham Population." *New England Journal of Medicine* 324(1991): 1839.

Long, P. "America's Top Food Myths." *Health* (October 1992):64.

Losonczy, K. G. et al. "Does Weight Loss from Middle Age to Old Age Explain the Inverse Weight Mortality in Old Age?" *American Journal of Epidemiology* 141(1995):312.

Lovelady, L. A. et al. "Effects of Exercise on Plasma Lipids and Metabolism of Lactating Women." *Medicine and Science in Sports and Exercise* 27(1995):22.

Lucas, A. R. et al. "50-year Trends in the Incidence of Anorexia Nervosa in Rochester, Minn.: A Population-Based Study." *American Journal of Psychiatry* 148(1991):917.

Maloney, M. J. et al. "Dieting Behavior and Eating Attitudes in Children." *Pediatrics* 84(1989):482.

Marano, H. E. *Style Is Not a Size.* New York: Bantam Books, 1991.

———. "Chemistry and Craving." *Psychology Today* (January/February 1993):30.

Marchi, M. et al. "Early Childhood Eating Behaviors and Adolescent Eating Disorders." *Journal of the American Academy of Child and Adolescent Psychiatry* 19(1990):112.

Martin, J. "Fitness Fun for the Whole Family." *American Health* (July/August 1995):70.

Martini, M. C. et al. "Effect of Menstrual Cycle on Energy and Nutrient Intake." *American Journal of Clinical Nutrition* 60(1994):895.

Matkovic, V. "Calcium and Primary Prevention of Osteoporosis." *Nutrition and the MD* 21(1995):1.

McBean, L. D. "Adolescent Nutrition: Issues and Challenges." *Dairy Council Digest* 58(1987):1.

McCann, J. B. et al. "The Eating Habits and Attitudes of Mothers of Children with Non-organic Failure to Thrive." *Archives of Disease in Childhood* 70(1994):234.

McKee, L. M. et al. "Genetic and Environmental Origins of Food Patterns." *Nutrition Today* (September/October 1990):26.

Mellin, L. M. et al. "Prevalance of Disordered Eating in Girls: A Survey of Middle Class Children." *Journal of the American Dietetic Association* 92(1992):851.

"Middle Age Spread." *Harvard Women's Health Watch* (August 1995):6.

Miller, A. et al. "Diets Incorporated." *Newsweek,* September 11, 1989, 56.

Miller, J. B. *Toward a New Psychology of Women,* 2nd ed. Boston: Beacon Press, 1986.

Miller, W. C. et al. "Diet Composition, Energy Intake, and Exercise in Relation to Body Fat in Men and Women." *American Journal of Clinical Nutrition* 52(1990):426.

Moore, D. C. "Body Image and Eating Behavior in Adolescent Girls." *American Journal of Diseases of Children.* 142(1988):1114.

"More on the Pitfalls of Television Watching." *Tufts University Diet and Nutrition Letter* 10(1992):6.

Morgan, J. et al. "Factors Discriminating Restrained and Unrestrained Eaters: A Retrospective Self-report Study." Unpublished ms., 1985.

Morris, A. et al. "The Changing Shape of Female Models." *International Journal of Eating Disorders* 8(1989):593.

Mortenson, G. M. et al. "Predictions of Body Satisfaction in College Women." *Journal of the American Dietetic Association* 93(1993):1037.

Moser, P. W. "Double Vision: Why Do We Never Match Up to Our Mind's Ideal?" *Self Magazine* (January 1989):51.

Moses, N. et al. "Fear of Obesity among Adolescent Girls." *Pediatrics* 83(1989):393.

Moss, R. A. et al. "Binge Eating, Vomiting, and Weight Fear in a Female High School Population." *Journal of Family Practice* 18(1984):313.

"Mother's Day Marathon." *Shape Magazine* (May 1995):129.

Murphy, A. S. et al. "Kindergarten Students' Food Preferences Are Not Consistent with Their Knowledge of the Dietary Guidelines." *Journal of the American Dietetic Association* 95(1995):219.

Napier, K. "Eggs." *American Health* (November 1995):75.

Nasser, M. "Culture and Weight Consciousness." *Journal of Psychosomatic Research* 32(1988):573.

Neumark-Sztainer, D. "Excessive Weight Preoccupation: Normative But Not Harmless." *Nutrition Today* 30(1995):68.

Neumark-Sztainer, D. et al. "Dieting and Binge Eating: Which Dieters Are at Risk?" *Journal of the American Dietetic Association* 95(1995):586.

"Newsbreaks: USDA Research Highlights." *Nutrition Today* 29(1994):4.

Nicklas, T. A. "Studies of Consistency of Dietary Intake during the First Four Years of Life in a Prospective Analysis: Bogalusa Heart Study." *Journal of the American College of Nutrition* 10(1991):254.

———. "Dietary Studies of Children: The Bogalusa Heart Study Experience." *Journal of the American Dietetic Association* 95(1995):1127.

Nidiffer, M. et al. "Attributes and Perceived Body Image of Students Seeking Nutrition Counseling in a University Wellness Program." *Journal of the American Dietetic Association* (Supplement) 92(1992):A-56.

"Nutrition and Your Health: Dietary Guidelines for Americans," 4th ed. US Department of Agriculture. US Department of Health and Human Services. Home and Garden Bulletin No. 232, 1995.

O'Neill, M. "So It May Be True After All—Eating Pasta Makes You Fat." *New York Times,* February 8, 1995, 1.

"Obesity: New Directions in Treatment." *Nutrition and the MD* 21(1995):1.

Olson, R. E. et al. "The Folly of Restricting Fat in the Diets of Children." *Nutrition Today* 30(1995):234.

Orbach, S. *Fat Is a Feminist Issue.* New York: Berkley Books, 1978.

Orenstein, P. *School Girls.* New York: Doubleday, 1994.

Palla, B. et al. "Medical Complications of Eating Disorders in Adolescents." *Pediatrics* 81(1988):613.

Palmer, R. L. et al. "Eating Disordered Patients Remember Their Parents: A Study Using the Parental-Bonding Instrument." *International Journal of Eating Disorders* 7(1988):101.

Patton, G. C. et al. "Abnormal Eating Attitudes in London Schoolgirls—A Prospective Epidemiological Study: Outcome at Twelve-month Follow-up." *Psychological Medicine* 20(1990):383.

Pazzaglia, G. et al. "Children's Television and Nutrition: Friends or Foes?" *Nutrition Today* 30(1995):6.

"Periscope." *Newsweek,* August 28, 1995, 8.

Pike, K. M. et al. "Mothers, Daughters, and Disordered Eating." *Journal of Abnormal Psychology* 100(1991):198.

Pipher, M. *Reviving Ophelia.* New York: Ballantine Books, 1994.

Polivy, J. et al. "Dieting and Bingeing." *American Psychologist* (February 1985):193.

———. "Undieting: A Program to Help People Stop Dieting." *International Journal of Eating Disorders* 11(1992):261.

Pomice, E. "When Kids Hate Their Bodies." *Redbook Magazine* (April 1995): 182.

Pope, H. G. et al. "Prevalence of Anorexia Nervosa and Bulimia in Three Student Populations." *International Journal of Eating Disorders* 3(1984):45.

Posner, B. M. et al. "Secular Trends in Diet and Risk Factors of Cardiovascular Disease: The Framingham Study." *Journal of the American Dietetic Association* 95(1995):171.

Potter, S. et al. "Does Infant Feeding Method Influence Maternal Postpartum Weight Loss?" *Journal of the American Dietetic Association* 91(1991):441.

Powell, J. J. et al. "The Effects of Different Percentages of Dietary Fat Intake, Exercise, and Caloric Restriction on Body Composition and Body Weight in Obese Women." *American Journal of Health Promotion* 8(1994):442.

Pugliese, M. T. et al. "Fear of Obesity: A Cause of Short Stature and Delayed Puberty." *New England Journal of Medicine* 309(1983): 513.

Rabinor, J. R. "Mother, Daughters and Eating Disorders: Honoring the Mother-Daughter Relationship." In Fallon, P., Katzman, M. A., and Wooley, S. C. *Feminist Perspectives on Eating Disorders.* New York: Guilford Press, 1994, p. 276.

Radcliffe, R. R. "What a New Study Reveals about Eating Disorders." *Shape Magazine* (October 1987):78.

Raitakari, O. T. et al. "Effects of Persistent Physical Activity on Coronary Risk Factors in Children and Young Adults." *American Journal of Epidemiology* 140(1994):195.

Rand, C. "Body Image in Contrast." *Shape Magazine* (October 1987):72.

Recker, R. R. et al. "Bone Gain in Young Adult Women." *Journal of the American Medical Association* 268(1992):2403.

Rich, A. *Of Woman Born.* New York: W. W. Norton, 1986.

Richards, M. H. et al. "Weight and Eating Concerns among Pre- and Young Adolescent Boys and Girls." *Journal of Adolescent Health Care* 11(1990): 203.

Rickard, K. A. et al. "The Play Approach to Learning in the Context of Families and Schools: An Alternative Paradigm for Nutrition and Fitness Education in the 21st Century." *Journal of the American Dietetic Association* 95(1995):1121.

Rittenbaugh, C. "Obesity as a Culture-bound Syndrome." *Culture, Medicine and Psychiatry* 6(1982):347.

Rodin, J. et al. "Women and Weight: A Normative Discontent." Nebraska Symposium on Motivation. Lincoln, Nebr.: University of Nebraska Press, 1984, p. 267.

Root, P. P. "Disordered Eating in Women of Color." *Sex Roles* 22(1990):525.

Rosen, J. C. et al. "Psychological Adjustment of Adolescents Attempting to Lose or Gain Weight." *Journal of Consulting and Clinical Psychology* 55(1987):742.

Rosen, L. W. et al. "Pathogenic Weight-control Behavior in Female Athletes." *The Physician and Sports Medicine* 14(1986):79.

Roughan, P. et al. "Long-term Effects of a Physiologically Based Group Programme for Women Preoccupied with Weight and Eating Behavior." *International Journal of Obesity* 14(1990):135.

Rubin, S. "Why Samoans Can't Figure Out America's Diet Mania." *San Francisco Chronicle,* July 6, 1982, 17.

Sabate, J. et al. "Lower Height of Lacto-ovovegetarian Girls at Preadolescence: An Indicator of Physical Maturation Delay?" *Journal of the American Dietetic Association* 92(1992):1263.

Sargent, J. D. et al. "Obesity and Stature in Adolescents and Earnings in Young Adulthood: Analysis of a British Cohort." *Archives of Pediatric and Adolescent Medicine* 148(1994):681.

Satter, E. *How to Get Your Kid to Eat . . . But Not Too Much.* Palo Alto, Calif.: Bull Publishing, 1987.

Schotte, D. E. et al. "Bulimia vs. Bulimic Behaviors on a College Campus." *Journal of the American Medical Association* 258(1987):1213.

"Second Time Around: Weight Study Gets Pounded." *Women's Health Advocate Newsletter* 2(1995):6.

Seligman, J. et al. "The Littlest Dieters." *Newsweek,* July 27, 1987, 48.

Serdula, M. K. et al. "Fruit and Vegetable Intake Among Adults in 16 States: Results of a Brief Telephone Survey." *American Journal of Public Health* 85(1995):236.

Shapiro, L. R. et al. "Obesity Prognosis: A Longitudinal Study of Children from the Age of 6 Months to 9 Years." *American Journal of Public Health* 74(1984):1968.

Shide, D. J. et al. "Information about the Fat Content of Preloads Influences Energy Intake in Healthy Women." *Journal of the American Dietetic Association* 95(1995):993.

Shisslak, C. M. et al. "Primary Prevention of Eating Disorders." *Journal of Consulting and Clinical Psychology* 55(1987):660.

Sigman-Grant, M. "Feeding Preschoolers: Balancing Nutritional and Developmental Needs." *Nutrition Today* (July/August 1992):13.

Silverstein, B. et al. "Possible Causes of the Thin Standard of Attractiveness for Women." *International Journal of Eating Disorders* 5(1986):907.

———. "Some Correlates of the Thin Standard of Bodily Attractiveness for Women." *International Journal of Eating Disorders* 5(1986):895.

Singleton, J. C. et al. "Role of Food and Nutrition in the Health Perceptions of Young Children." *Journal of the American Dietetic Association* 92(1992): 68.

Slap, G. B. et al. *Teenage Health Care.* New York: Pocket Books, 1994.

"Smart Students, Foolish Choices." *Tufts University Diet and Nutrition Letter.* 11(1993):2.

Smith, D. E. et al. "Longitudinal Changes in Adiposity Associated with Pregnancy." *Journal of the American Medical Association* 271(1994):1747.

Smolak, L. et al. "Separation-Individuation Difficulties and the Distinction between Bulimia Nervosa and Anorexia Nervosa in College Women." *International Journal of Eating Disorders* 14(1993):33.

Somer, E. "Crank It Up." *Shape Magazine* (October 1994):62.

Sorensen, T. I. A. et al. "Childhood Body Mass Index—Genetic and Familial Environmental Influences Assessed in a Longitudinal Study." *International Journal of Obesity* 16(1992):705.

St. Jeor, S. T. "The Role of Weight Management in the Health of Women." *Journal of the American Dietetic Association* 93(1993):1007.

Stallings, S. et al. "Normal Weight Women." *Shape Magazine* (January 1990): 34.

Steiger, H. et al. "Defense Styles and Parental Bonding in Eating-disordered Women." *International Journal of Eating Disorders* 8(1989):131.

———. "Personality and Family Disturbances in Eating Disorder Patients: Comparison of 'Restricters' and 'Bingers' to Normal Controls." *International Journal of Eating Disorders* 10(1991):501.

———. "Personality and Family Features of Adolescent Girls with Eating Symptoms: Evidence for Restricter/Binger Differences in a Nonclinical Population." *Addictive Behaviors* 16(1991):303.

Stein, A. et al. "Children of Mothers with Bulimia Nervosa." *British Medical Journal* 299(1989):777.

———. "An Observation Study of Mothers with Eating Disorders and Their Infants." *Journal of Child Psychology* 35(1993):733.

Steinem, G. *Revolution from Within: A Book of Self-Esteem.* Boston: Little, Brown, 1992.

Steiner-Adair, C. "The Body Politic: Normal Adolescent Development and the Development of Eating Disorders." *Journal of the Academy of Psychoanalysis* 14(1986):95.

Stephenson, M. G. et al. "The 1985 NHIS Findings: Nutrition Knowledge and Baseline Data for the Weight Loss Objectives." *Public Health Reports* 102(1987):61.

Stern, S. L. et al. "Family Environment in Anorexia Nervosa and Bulima." *International Journal of Eating Disorders* 8(1989):25.

Sternlieb, J. J. et al. "A Survey of Health Problems, Practices, and Needs of Youth." *Pediatrics* 49(1972):177.

Stevens, J. et al. "Attitudes towards Body Size and Dieting: Differences between Elderly Black and White Women." *American Journal of Public Health* 84(1994):1322.

Story, M. et al. "Demographic and Risk Factors Associated with Chronic Dieting in Adolescents." *American Journal of Diseases of Children* 145(1991): 994.

———. "Weight Perceptions and Weight Control Practices in American Indian and Alaska Native Adolescents: A National Survey." *Archives of Pediatric and Adolescent Health* 148(1994):567.

Strasberger, V. C. "Does Television Affect Learning and School Performance?" *Pediatrics* 13(1986):141.

Striegel-Moore, R. et al. "Psychological and Behavioral Correlates of Feeling Fat in Women." *International Journal of Eating Disorders* 5(1986):935.

———. "Toward an Understanding of Risk Factors in Bulimia." *American Psychologist* 41(1986):246.

Strober, M. et al. "Familial Contributions to the Etiology and Course of Anorexia Nervosa and Bulimia." *Journal of Consulting and Clinical Psychology* 55(1987):654.

Stunkard, A. J. et al. "The Three-factor Eating Questionnaire to Measure Dietary Restraint, Disinhibition, and Hunger." *Journal of Psychosomatic Research* 29(1985):71.

Sylvester, G. P. et al. "Children's Television and Nutrition: Friends or Foes?" *Nutrition Today* 30(1995):6.

Telsh, C. F. et al. "The Effects of a Very Low Calorie Diet on Binge Eating." *Behavior Therapy* 24(1993):177.

Ternus, M. "Sugar and Kids: Not Necessarily a Dastardly Duo." *Environmental Nutrition* 14(1991):1.

Thompson, J. K. "Larger than Life." *Psychology Today* (April 1986):38.

Thompson, J. K. et al. "Body Shape Preferences: Effects in Instructional Protocol and Level of Eating Disturbance." *International Journal of Eating Disorders* 10(1991):193.

Thorton, B. et al. "Gender Role Typing, the Superwoman Ideal and the Potential for Eating Disorders." *Sex Roles* 25(1991):469.

Tienboon, P. et al. "Adolescent Perceptions of Body Weight and Parents' Weight for Height Status." *Journal of Adolescent Health* 15(1994): 263.

Timko, C. et al. "Femininity/Masculinity and Disordered Eating in Women: How Are They Related?" *International Journal of Eating Disorders* 6(1987): 701.

Tucker, S. "What Is the Ideal Body?" *Shape Magazine* (July 1990):95.

"TV Food Ads Feed Kids the Wrong Messages." *Tufts University Diet and Nutrition Letter* 12(1995):7.

Urbanska, W. "The Body Image Report." *Shape Magazine* (March 1994):73.

U.S. Bureau of the Census. *Statistical Abstract of the United States,* 110th ed. Washington, D.C.: U.S. Government Printing Office, 1991.

Vandereycken, W. et al. "Siblings of Patients with Eating Disorders." *International Journal of Eating Disorders* 12(1992):273.

Van Gaal, L. et al. "Lipid and Lipoprotein Changes after Long-term Weight Reduction: The Influence of Gender and Body Fat Distribution." *Journal of the American College of Nutrition* 14(1995):382.

van Wezel-Meijler, G. et al. "The Offspring of Mothers with Anorexia Nervosa: A High Risk Group of Undernutrition and Stunting?" *European Journal of Pediatrics* 149(1989):130.

Vickers, M. J. "Understanding Obesity in Women." *Journal of Obstetric Gynecologic and Neonatal Nursing* (January/February 1993):17.

"Vital Statistics." *Health Magazine* (March/April 1993):12.

Wadden, T. A. et al. "Dissatisfaction with Weight and Figure in Obese Girls: Discontent but Not Depression." *International Journal of Obesity* 13(1989): 89.

Waller, G. et al. "Family Adaptability and Cohesion: Relation to Eating Attitudes and Disorders." *International Journal of Eating Disorders* 9(1990): 225.

———. "Who Knows Best? Family Interaction and Eating Disorders." *British Journal of Psychiatry* 156(1990):546.

Wardle, J. et al. "Adolescent Concerns about Weight and Eating: A Social-Developmental Perspective." *Journal of Psychosomatic Research* 34(1990): 377.

———. "Control and Loss of Control over Eating: An Experimental Investigation." *Journal of Abnormal Psychology* 94(1988):78.

———. "Culture and Body Image: Body Perception and Weight Concern in Young Asian and Caucasian British Women." *Journal of Community and Applied Social Psychology* 3(1993):173.

"Warning: Keep Dieting Out of Reach of Children." *Tufts University Diet and Nutrition Letter* 11(1993):3.

Warwick, Z. S. "Development of Taste Preferences: Implications for Nutrition and Health." *Nutrition Today* (March/April 1990):15.

Watson, T. et al. "Are You Too Fat?" *US News & World Report,* January 8, 1996, 52.

Webb, D. "Does Pasta Make You Fat?" *American Health* (October 1995):80.

Webb, M. "Our Daughters, Ourselves." *Ms. Magazine* (November/December 1992):30.

Wertheim, E. H. et al. "Psychosocial Predictors of Weight Loss and Binge Eating in Adolescent Girls and Boys." *International Journal of Eating Disorders* 12(1991):151.

"When Growing Pains Hurt Too Much: Teens at Risk." *Tufts University Diet and Nutrition Letter* 6(1991):3.

Whisenent, S. L. et al. "Eating Disorders: Current Nutrition Therapy and Perceived Needs in Dietetics Education and Research." *Journal of the American Dietetic Association* 95(1995):1109.

Whitaker, A. et al. "The Struggle to Be Thin: A Survey of Anorexic and Bulimic Symptoms on a Non-referred Adolescent Population." *Psychological Medicine* 19(1989):143.

White, J. H. "Feminism, Eating, and Mental Health." *Advances in Nursing Science* 13(1991):68.

Willett, W. C. et al. "Weight, Weight Change, and Coronary Heart Disease in Women." *Journal of the American Medical Association* 273(1995):461.

Williams, L. "Stalking the Elusive Healthy Diet." *New York Times,* October 11, 1995, C1.

Williamson, D. F. et al. "The 10-year Incidence of Overweight and Major Weight Gain in US Adults." *Archives of Internal Medicine* 150(1990):665.

———. "Weight Loss Attempts in Adults: Goals, Duration, and Rate of Weight Loss." *American Journal of Public Health* 82(1992): 1251.

Wing, R. R. et al. "Effect of Modest Weight Loss on Changes in Cardiovascular Risk Factors: Are There Differences between Men and Women or between Weight Loss and Maintenance?" *International Journal of Obesity* 19(1995): 67.

Wood, M. "Weight Loss: A Sex-linked Trait." *Agricultural Research* (August 1995):14.

Woodward, D. R. "What Sort of Teenager Has Low Intakes of Energy Nutrients?" *British Journal of Nutrition* 53(1985):241.

Wooley, O. W. et al. "The Beverly Hills Eating Disorder: The Mass Marketing of Anorexia Nervosa." *International Journal of Eating Disorders* 1(1982): 57.

Wooley, S. C. "A Woman's Body in a Man's World." *Shape Magazine* (October 1987):70.

Wooley, S. C. et al. "Feeling Fat in a Thin Society." *Glamour Magazine* (February 1984):198.